A DENTAL PRACTITIONER HANDBOOK
SERIES EDITED BY DONALD D. DERRICK, D.D.S., L.D.S., R.C.S.

CRANIOFACIAL EMBRYOLOGY

GEOFFREY H. SPERBER
B.Sc.(Hons), B.D.S., M.S., Ph.D.

*Professor of Oral Biology, Faculty of Dentistry,
University of Alberta, Edmonton, Canada*

With a Foreword by
PHILLIP V. TOBIAS
F.R.S.S.Af., F.L.S., F.R.A.I., M.B.B.Ch., Ph.D., D.Sc.

*Dean of the Faculty of Medicine and
Head of Department of Anatomy, University of the Witwatersrand*

Third Edition

WRIGHT · PSG
BRISTOL   LONDON   BOSTON
1981

Published by
John Wright & Sons Ltd, 42–44 Triangle West, Bristol BS8 1EX.
England
John Wright PSG Inc., 545 Great Road, Littleton, Massachusetts 01460, U.S.A.

First edition,	1973
Second edition,	1976
Japanese edition,	1976
Third edition,	1981

British Library Cataloguing in Publication Data

Sperber, Geoffrey
    Craniofacial embryology,—
3rd ed.—(A Dental practitioner handbook; no. 15)
    1. Embryology, Human
    2. Head
    3. Dentistry
    I. Title   II. Series
    616'.64   QM611

ISBN 0 7236 0552 1

PRINTED IN GREAT BRITAIN BY HENRY LING LTD, A SUBSIDIARY OF
JOHN WRIGHT AND SONS LTD, AT THE DORSET PRESS, DORCHESTER

PREFACE TO THE THIRD EDITION

THE call for a third edition of this book within seven years of its first appearance confirms that craniofacial ontogeny is an established subject of concern to practitioners of orofacial therapy. The development of the craniofacial complex is occupying an increasingly important role in undergraduate curricula of medical, dental and speech therapy programmes, and is becoming an essential requirement for postgraduate courses in orthodontics and craniofacial surgery.

When this book was first written in 1973, most known aspects of craniofacial embryology could be reviewed within the compass of a compact text. Since then the subject has so burgeoned that in a short book even an overview of the torrents of research reports is a difficult task and representation of every perspective, ranging from molecular biology to therapeutic considerations of anomalous development, a near impossibility.

Errors of fact and judgement made in previous editions have been corrected, but despite the virtual re-writing of this book, errors must surely have entered this edition as readily as they were removed from the others. My concern is not only to present conventional concepts, but to prepare neophytes for new directions of ontogenetic investigation. Each successive advance in understanding the development of the craniofacial complex reveals new problems that make complete knowledge ever further from attainment.

The recent spectacular advances in scanning electron microscopy that have been applied to the developing embryo have yielded dramatic photographs of various stages of development. The privileged inclusion of such photographs in this new edition adds stunning evidence to the wonders of morphogenesis that verbal description can never attain.

Nearly every chapter has been revised in the light of new knowledge. The text has been expanded to follow some aspects of postnatal growth, particularly of the maxillofacial complex, to increase the clinical application of this study. The initial aim of a simplified presentation has, on occasion, necessitated the procrustean fitting of conflicting hypotheses into a single conceptual bed. Where

v

conflicts are evident, it is hoped that they might stimulate the reader to resolve the uncertainties.

Many new illustrations have been added to this third edition and previous illustrations have been revised for better comprehension. It is hoped that this expanded edition will continue to facilitate comprehension of normal craniofacial anatomy and its developmental defects in a succinct manner without overwhelming the reader by their complexity.

Edmonton, 1981   G.H.S.

PREFACE TO THE FIRST EDITION

THE length of dental undergraduate education has remained essentially unchanged ever since the formalization of university dental training. Despite this rigid time limitation, an enormous increase in the amount of material that is required to be presented and understood by the dental student has occurred in recent years. It has become necessary to select carefully 'relevant' material for good dental practice from the *embarras de richess* of knowledge currently available, so that it can be reasonably accommodated within the traditional five-year undergraduate dental curriculum. Among the 'basic science' subjects, the one that has suffered most from pruning of the undergraduate curriculum has been anatomy, and in particular, developmental anatomy, to the extent that embryology is now allocated a very minor portion of the restricted teaching time made available to anatomy in most dental schools. Yet, paradoxically, increasing emphasis is being placed upon the treatment of developmental defects in current medicine and dentistry, which is exemplified in the latter case by the rising demand for treatment of dentofacial deformities.

An adequate understanding of normal development is necessary for knowledgeable handling of abnormal development, and, to this end, this text is devoted to a rather detailed examination of craniofacial growth and development. The vast majority of embryology textbooks are designed for medical students, with little emphasis on craniofacial development which is so relevant to the dental student, and on which subject emphasis is particularly required for orthodontic teaching. On the other hand, those textbooks devoted to 'dental embryology' neglect the initial stages of total embryological development, and often fail to indicate the clinical implications of maldevelopment of the interlocking craniofacial constituents.

This book, dealing with craniofacial development, has been designed to fill an obvious hiatus in dental education. It is an account of craniofacial growth starting at the beginning of embryonic development. This may prove tedious to those interested in the surgery and mechano-therapy of dentofacial orthopaedics, but I believe it is necessary to gain a full understanding of the numerous components of craniofacial structure in order to intervene successfully in their complex interactions during their development. An attempt has been made to select those parts of early development that are of greatest concern to craniofacial growth, and to highlight those features that would be of interest and importance to the dentist. For this reason, most of the extracranial components of embryonic development have been excluded from this description.

Craniofacial growth is a field of extraordinarily divergent views, with many hypotheses offered to explain observed phenomena. This book is an attempt to reconcile many of these views with the object of simplifying as far as possible an extremely complex set of events.

Wherever possible, the impact of the complex developmental and growth phenomena of the dentofacial complex upon clinical practice has been indicated. An understanding of the causes and mechanisms of developmental defects should result in knowledgeable evaluation, treatment, and prognostication of maldevelopment of the orofacial complex. To this purpose is this book dedicated.

G.H.S.

ACKNOWLEDGEMENTS

To my colleagues, whose inspiration and ideas are woven into the fabric of this book, I wish to express my warm appreciation. I am particularly indebted to Professor P. V. Tobias, Head of the Department of Anatomy, University of the Witwatersrand, Johannesburg for writing the Foreword, to Professor J. W. Osborn, Head of the Department of Oral Biology, to Dr R. D. Haryett, Orthodontist, and to Dr G. W. Thompson, Dean of the Faculty of Dentistry, University of Alberta, Edmonton, for helpful suggestions.

My gratitude is expressed to Mrs Elise Duggan for her skilful portrayal of developing morphology, and to Mr Edison MacQuarrie for his expert photographic contributions.

My thanks go to the authors and publishers of diagrams and photographs that are acknowledged in the captions for permission to include their copyright publications in this work. I am most grateful to Professor Dr E. Blechschmidt and Dr R. Gasser for providing the photographs of *Figs. 26–31* to Professor Hideo Nishimura for photographs from his *Atlas of Prenatal Development of the Human with Special Reference to Craniofacial Structures*, to Dr Rainer-Reginald Miethke for *Figs. 111* and *112* from his text *Zur intrauterinen Entwicklung der Kiefer und Lippen bei menschlichen Feten*, Verlag 'Die Quintessenz' W. Berlin, and to W. B. Saunders Co., Philadelphia for *Fig. 105*.

I wish to express my deep gratitude to my wife, Robyn, and Heather, Jacqueline and Steven for their forbearance during the preparation of this work, and for the time devoted to its writing that should rightfully have been theirs.

The friendly cooperation of John Wright & Sons Ltd is most gratefully acknowledged in their publication of this book.

And surely we are all out of the computation of our age, and every man is some months elder than he bethinks him; for we live, move, have a being, and are subject to the actions of the elements, and the malice of diseases, in that other World, the truest Microcosm, the Womb of our Mother.

SIR THOMAS BROWNE: *Religio Medici*, 1642

CONTENTS

xi

FOREWORD

By Professor P. V. Tobias

EVER since Leonardo da Vinci measured a series of embryos and fetuses of different ages, the story of development before birth has fascinated countless students. It is truly a remarkable tale of an orderly sequence of events, by which each human being blossoms out from a minute egg cell, one fifty-thousand-millionth of the weight of an adult man. Thus, descriptive embryology can be studied for its own sake. We can, however, probe more deeply and ask: How do the changes occur? Are they, as Dobzhansky has remarked, simply a matter of assimilation of transformed groceries? Or is there more to it than that? Indeed, in its experimental and causal approach, embryology is rapidly becoming one of the most advanced vistas of modern cellular and molecular biology.

If only time would allow each of us to dawdle for a while and admire the view on this exciting side-track!

Instead, for most of those who read this book, experimental and molecular embryology is a glimpse from the window of a railway carriage—in focus for a moment, then gone, as one rushes on to other destinations.

Of more immediate relevance to dental students is the help that embryology may give to an understanding of normal anatomy.

A knowledge of development is a precious key to a grasp of the anatomical finished products. Although this principle holds for all parts of the body, it is probably true to say that it is most valid for the head and neck. Generations of dental and medical students have been challenged and perplexed by the intricacies of fine morphological detail in this area. They have toiled with the structural complexities of the teeth and their supporting tissues, of the mouth, nose, throat, and larynx, of the brain and those parts of the head related to the special senses, to the postural control of the head on the neck and spine, to the cranial nerves, the salivary glands, the speech mechanism—and the highways and byways which connect brain and head to trunk.

It is therefore something of a relief to learn how much embryonic development can help one to gain an insight into the apparently involved structural make-up of the head. What had looked like an appalling burden on the students' memory is seen as a superbly logical plan, an obvious and inevitable pattern. Given the formative pathways—and the anatomy must follow as night follows day. Almost miraculously, the egg is unscrambled—and memory and understanding are nourished in the process.

This is true for the study of anatomical variations and congenital malformations, no less than of normal anatomy. How else can one fathom cleft palates, underdeveloped jaws, too many—or too few—teeth, very large tongues or very small mouths: except as the end-results of lines of development different in some or other respect from the normal pathways? So the embryological approach may clarify many of the hundreds of congenital variations in the head and neck. It is a vital key to the mastery of the aberrant—as well as of the normal.

It is because of his deep conviction that this approach is valuable, even invaluable, that Professor Geoffrey Sperber has written this little textbook. It represents a sincere attempt to make the life of the dental student and graduate easier: by opening up to them the advantages and the delights of the developmental way of learning things. With Professor Sperber's dual background of dentistry and anatomy, he is well placed to achieve this objective. His meticulous attention to detail, coupled with a clear appreciation of the sign-posts leading through the maze of items, has led him to provide an extremely useful text, of a pioneering kind. This is a book from which undergraduate and graduate students of dentistry and oral medicine should derive great benefit. In a word, it is an introduction to the embryology, the morphology, and the teratology of the masticatory apparatus—and of the head built around it. As such, its readers should find it falling into the third of the three classes to which Francis Bacon allotted all books, when he wrote (*Of Studies*):—

> '*Some books are to be tasted, others to be swallowed, and some few to be chewed and digested.*'

SECTION I

GENERAL EMBRYOLOGY

I will praise Thee: for I am fearfully and wonderfully made.

Psalm CXXXIX 14,

The student of Nature wonders the more and is astonished the less, the more conversant he becomes with her operations, but of all the perennial miracles she offers to his inspection, perhaps the most worthy of admiration is the development of a plant or animal from its embryo.

Huxley

1

CHAPTER 1

THE STOMATOGNATHIC COMPLEX

THE mouth serves as a focal point of interest to more medical and dental specialties than any other single part of the body. It is of concern to the anaesthetist in gaining access to the respiratory system. It is within the domains of the otorhinolaryngologist and of the maxillofacial, the plastic, and the oral surgeon. It is the very special territory of the speech therapist, and an area of much significance to the nutritionist, dermatologist, haematologist, and allergist. The expressions portrayed by the mouth are subject to the scrutiny of the psychiatrist. Above all, as it contains the masticatory system, it is the pre-eminent field of interest of the dental profession and all its sub-specialties.

The buccal cavity not only serves as a portal of entry to the gastrointestinal system, but, being also the source of vocal communication, is, in a very real sense, the mouthpiece of emotional expression. This is true not only for the articulation of words, but also in determining facial demeanour. Smiling, grinning, grimacing, pouting, scowling, and gnashing of teeth are all oral manifestations of various moods. The mouth is believed to be the first organ of which consciousness is aware. The mouth serves from birth onwards as the fount of emotional satisfaction in satiating hunger and slaking thirst for self-preservation, and expressing and receiving erotic stimuli by osculatory activities as a prelude to reproduction. It is small wonder that dental malocclusion and deformities of the orofacial complex are of major significance not only to dental health but also to mental health and social well-being.

The masticatory apparatus, comprising the dentition, the jaws, and the face in which it is housed and which it helps constitute, is a constantly altering entity, although its rate of change varies considerably at different periods of life. This alteration of dentofacial form is the result of many interacting factors influencing the hard and soft tissues that constitute the head, face, and masticatory apparatus. The developmental ontogeny of the dentofacial complex is dependent primarily upon the following three elements:—

1. *Genetic endowment* $\begin{cases} \text{Inherited genotype} \\ \text{Operation of genetic mechanisms} \end{cases}$

2. *Environmental factors* $\begin{cases} \text{Nutrition and biochemical interactions} \\ \text{Physical phenomena—temperature,} \\ \text{pressures, hydration, etc.} \end{cases}$

3. *Functional forces*   { Extrinsic and intrinsic forces of muscle actions, space-occupying organs and cavities, and growth expansion.

Three basic types of tissue constitute the dentofacial form:—

1. *Dental tissues:* Enamel, dentine, cementum, pulp, and periodontal ligament.
2. *Skeletal tissues:* Bone, cartilage, and ligaments.
3. *Soft tissues:*
    a. Neuromuscular:
        i. Perioral (facial) muscles.
        ii. Intraoral (masticatory and tongue) muscles.
    b. Tissues other than muscle: i.e., epithelia, glands, circulatory tissue, mucous membranes, connective tissues, etc.

The arrangement of these three basic varieties of tissues is of concern to the dentist, and is dependent upon the operation of the three functional elements enumerated above, the activities of which are largely beyond his control. By fully appreciating and understanding the natural forces acting upon and influencing the teeth from the time of their initiation to the time of their full eruption and utilization, the dentist can better manipulate the dentition with factors that he *can* control in attaining an ideal occlusion. Careful and calculated intervention of a fourth element, maxillofacial surgery or orthodontic forces, including preventive and interceptive procedures designed to operate within the context of the three natural determinants of dentofacial form, will result in successful guidance of developmental malocclusions towards a desired conformation of the dentition and jaws.

The morphological traits of individual bones may be genetically determined, but their subsequent development and orientation to one another may be influenced by their environment. Orthodontic forces cannot alter the morphogenetic growth patterns of individual bones; they can only alter the relationships between the various bones making up the craniofacial complex. Orthodontic or surgical therapy is most potent in altering the relationship of teeth to one another in their bony and soft-tissue setting.

Mastication is but one of the many functions carried out by the orofacial structures; breathing and speech, gustation and deglutition, olfaction, facial expression, and even hearing and vision are part of the functions of the orofacial complex. Each of these functions is served by a set of organs and tissues which constitute a 'functional matrix', and their presence and actions influence the configuration of the face and jaws. The concept of 'functional matrices' involves consideration of the presence and functioning of various soft tissues and organs as forming influences upon bone development and morphology. Thus, muscles attaching to bones, the eyes, the brain, neurovascular triads, the tongue, and other soft tissues exert a shaping influence upon bones and joints. Distinction is made between *periosteal matrices* that attach to and remodel bone, exemplified by muscles and ligaments, and *capsular matrices* that enclose masses or spaces, exemplified by organs contiguous with bone, and displace bones by their enlargement. Volumetric expansion of the oronasopharyngeal functioning spaces greatly influences facial bone development. The intervention of artificial forces, such as is the practice in orthodontic therapy, may constitute a 'functional matrix' designed to direct growth or odontoskeletal relationships into a desired configuration.

The development and interaction of the many 'functional matrices' present in the dento-orognathofacial complex determines in various ways the positions of the teeth and jaws and the occlusal patterns established by them. The developing fetal and infant mouth is not merely a smaller and less accomplished version of the adult mouth, but is a qualitatively different structure, with constantly changing organizational rules of growth, differentiation and behavioural characteristics.

Anomalies of development of the orofacial complex are of increasing concern to the health professions. Dental malocclusions, cleft palates and lips and the like are reflections of genetic endowment, which, because they are being treated, allow for their perpetuation in progeny in ever-increasing numbers. Between 20 and 60 per cent of North American children, depending upon the criteria used, display malocclusion of the teeth and jaws. An understanding of orofacial development is essential to an understanding of malocclusion.

SELECTED BIBLIOGRAPHY

BOSMA, J. F. (1972), 'Form and Function in the Infant's Mouth and Pharynx', Chapt. 1 in *Third Symposium on Oral Sensation and Perception* (Ed. BOSMA, J. F.). Springfield, Ill.: Thomas.

BROADBENT, B. H., Sr., BROADBENT, B. H., Jr., and GOLDEN, W. H. (1975) *Bolton Standards of Dentofacial Developmental Growth.* St. Louis: Mosby.

CRELIN, E. S. (1973), *Functional Anatomy of the Newborn.* New Haven: Yale University Press.

ENLOW, D. H. (1975), *Handbook of Facial Growth.* Philadelphia: Saunders.

HIRSCHFELD, W. J. (1970), 'Time Series and Exponential Smoothing Methods applied to the Analysis and Prediction of Growth', *Growth,* **34,** 129.

HOOLEY, J. R. (1967), 'The Infant's Mouth', *J. Am. dent. Ass.,* **75,** 95.

HOUPT, M. I. (1970), 'Growth of the Cranio-facial Complex of the Human Fetus', *Am. J. Orthod.,* **58,** 373.

KROGMAN, W. M. (1968), 'Biological Timing and the Dento-facial Complex', *J. Dent. Child.*, **35**, 175, 328, 377.
— — (1973), 'Craniofacial Growth and Development', *J. Am. dent. Ass.*, **87**, 1037.
MOSS, M. L. (1962), 'The Functional Matrix', in *Vistas in Orthodontics* (Ed. KRAUS, B. S., and RIEDEL, R. A.). Philadelphia: Lea & Febiger.
— — (1971), *Functional Cranial Analysis and the Functional Matrix.* Proceedings of the Conference on Patterns of Orofacial Growth and Development. Report No. 6. Washington: American Speech and Hearing Association.
— — (1972), 'An Introduction to the Neurobiology of Orofacial Growth', *Acta Biotheor.*, **21**, 236.
NEPOLA, S. R. (1969), 'The Intrinsic and Extrinsic Factors influencing the Growth and Development of the Jaws: Heredity and Functional Matrix', *Am. J. Orthod.*, **55**, 499.
SCOTT, J. H. (1967), *Dento-facial Development and Growth.* Oxford: Pergamon.
SINCLAIR, D. (1978), *Human Growth after Birth*, 3rd Ed. London: Oxford University Press.
VAN LIMBORGH, J. (1970), 'A New View on the Control of the Morphogenesis of the Skull', *Acta morph. neerl.-scand.*, **8**, 143.
— — (1972), 'The Role of Genetic and Local Environmental Factors in the Control of Postnatal Craniofacial Morphogenesis', *Ibid.*, **10**, 37.
WALKER, G. F. (1972), 'A New Approach to the Analysis of Craniofacial Morphology and Growth', *Am. J. Orthod.*, **61**, 221.

CHAPTER 2

EARLY EMBRYONIC DEVELOPMENT

*Over the structure of the cell rises the structure of
plants and animals, which exhibit the yet more
complicated, elaborate combinations of millions and
billions of cells coordinated and differentiated in
the most extremely different ways.*

HERTWIG

THE mating of male and female gametes in the maternal uterine tube
initiates the development of a *zygote*—the first identification of an
individual. The union of the haploid number of chromosomes (23)
of each gamete confers the hereditary material of each parent upon
the newly established diploid number of chromosomes (46) of the
zygote. All the inherited characteristics of an individual and its
sex are thereby established at the time of union of the gametes. The
single totipotential cell of approximately 140 μm. diameter resulting
from the union very soon commences mitotic division to produce
a rapidly increasing number of smaller-sized cells, so that the 16-cell
stage, known as the *morula*, is not much larger than the initial
zygote. These cells of the early zygote reveal no significant outward
differences of form. However, the chromosomes of these cells
must necessarily contain the potential for differentiation of subsequent cell generations into the variety of cell forms that later constitute the different tissues of the body. The genetic material contained
in the re-constituted diploid number of 46 chromosomes of the initial
zygote cell, by replication, is identical to that to be found in its
progeny. The activity of this replicated genetic material would,
however, vary as the subsequent cell generations departed from the
archetype 'primitive' cell. Parts of the genetic material would be
active at certain stages of development, while other parts might
remain quiescent at those particular times of development, only
to become active at others. Proliferation of the cells of the zygote
allows expression of their potential for differentiation into the great
variety of cell types that constitute the different tissues of the body.
The differentiation of these early pluripotential cells into specialized
forms is dependent upon genetic, cytoplasmic, and environmental
factors that act at critical times during their proliferation and growth.

Differentiation

The transformation of the ovum into a full-fledged organism, by
which process there is an orderly enlargement and diversification of

7

the proliferating cells of the morula, is the result of the selective activation and repression of the diploid set of genes carried in each cell. Which one of a pair of gene alleles contained in the diploid set of autosomal chromosomes is expressed depends on their similarity (homozygosity) or dissimilarity (heterozygosity). In the latter case, the degree of dominance or recessiveness of each allele of the pair determines the phenotypic expression of the gene. The expression of the traits governed by genes on the pair of non-autosomal or sex chromosomes is somewhat different. In females there is inactivation of one of the two X chromosomes and failure of expression of its genes (the Lyon hypothesis). In the male the presence of the Y chromosome and only a single X chromosome accounts for the sex-linkage of certain inherited traits.

A programmed sequence of development known as *epigenesis* occurs and is dependent upon *determination* that restricts multipotentiality, and *differentiation* of proliferating cells. These developmental events result from continuous interactions between cells and their microenvironments. As a consequence of differentiation, new varieties of cell types and tissues develop that interact with one another by *induction*, producing an increasingly complex organism. Induction alters the developmental course of responsive tissues, whose capacity to react is known as *competence*, to produce different tissues from which organs and systems arise. Inductive interactions may take place in several ways in different tissues. Interactions may occur by direct cellular contact, or may be mediated by diffusible agents, or even by inductors enclosed in vesicles. The mechanisms involved in these processes include gene activation and inactivation, protein translation mechanics, varying cell membrane selectivities, intercellular adhesions and repulsions and cell migration that produce precise cell positioning. Cell position is a key factor in early morphogenesis, since microenvironments activate or inhibit mechanisms leading to cellular diversification. All these events are critically timed and are under hormonal, metabolic and nutritional influences. The biochemical foundations of these complex functions, and the nature and manner of operation of their controlling factors, are at present little understood and are among the central challenges of contemporary biology. This compendium of manifold biochemical reactions leads to *cytodifferentiation* and *histodifferentiation*, resulting in the formation of epithelial and mesenchymal tissues that acquire specialized structure and function (*Fig. 1*). Epithelial–mesenchymal interactions that provide for reciprocal cell differentiation are essential prerequisites for *organogenesis* that results in organs and systems being produced (*Fig. 2*).

The entire group of above processes are marvellously integrated to form the external and internal configuration of the embryo,

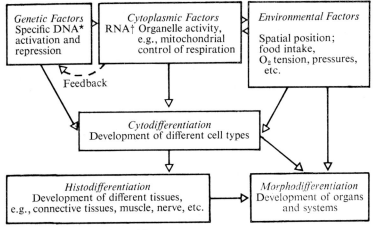

*DNA: Deoxyribonucleic acid.
†RNA: Ribonucleic acid.

Fig. 1.

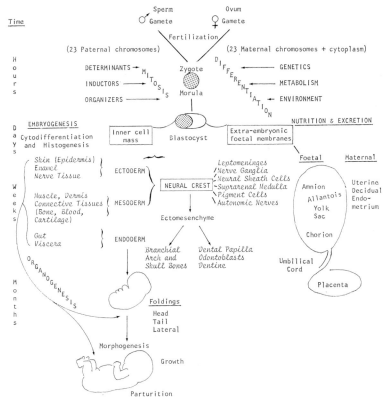

Fig. 2. Schematized synopsis of salient features of general embryology.

constituting *morphogenesis*, the process of development of form and size, that determines the morphology of organs, systems and the whole body. Not only is mitosis and cell growth essential for embryonic development, but, paradoxically, even cell death—genetically and hormonally controlled—forms a significant part of normal embryogenesis. By means of programmed cell death, tissues and organs useful only during embryonic life, and phylogenetic vestiges developed during ontogeny are eliminated.

The expressed character of differentiated cells (the phenotype) will depend firstly on their genetic constitution (the genotype) and, secondly, on the type and degree of gene expression and repression and environmental influence that has taken place during differentiation. Defective genes (mutations) or abnormal chromosome numbers (aneuploidy or polyploidy) will pattern aberrant development. Adverse environmental factors, both prenatal and postnatal, can deviate the genotypic pattern from normal development. Neither heredity (the genotype) nor the environment ever work exclusively in patterning development, but always in combination to produce the phenotype.

Disturbances of the inductive patterns of embryonic tissues will result in congenital defects of development. *Teratology* constitutes the study of such abnormal development. Malformations of the face and jaws are frequently part of congenital abnormality syndromes that may be amenable to surgical, orthopaedic, orthodontic and therapeutic correction.

Growth

Growth is a fundamental attribute of developing organisms. The dramatic increase in size that characterizes the living embryo is a consequence of: (1) An increase in the number of cells resulting from mitotic divisions (hyperplasia); (2) An increase in the size of the individual cells (hypertrophy); and (3) An increase in the amount of non-cellular material. Hyperplasia tends to predominate in the early embryo, while hypertrophy largely prevails in its later enlargement. Once differentiation of a tissue has been established, further development is predominantly that of growth. The rate of growth of a tissue is inherently determined, but is, of course, also dependent upon environmental conditions. The health, diet, race and sex of an individual influence the rate and extent of growth.

Growth may be *interstitial*, where increase in bulk occurs within a tissue or organ, or *appositional*, where surface deposition of tissue enlarges its size. Interstitial growth characterizes soft tissues, while hard tissues (bone, dental tissues) necessarily increase by apposition.

Growth is not merely an increase in size. If it were, the embryo would expand like a balloon, and the adult would simply be an

10

enlarged fetus. The resulting unproportioned growth would produce a grossly distorted adult with a head as large as the rest of the body. Not all tissues, organs or parts develop at the same rate, since *differential* growth accounts for a varying proportioned increase in size. The head is precocious in its development, constituting half the body size in the fetus (*see Frontispiece*), but later undergoing a relative decrease in relation to total body size. Each organ system grows at its own predetermined rate, accounting for proportional discrepancies in size at different periods of life. Some organ systems enlarge precociously and, subsequently, remain nearly stationary in size, while others continue to grow until adolescence. The lymphoid system (tonsils, thymus, etc.), after extremely rapid growth in early childhood, even regresses in size before adulthood (*Fig. 3*).

Increments in growth are constantly changing with chronological age, being most rapid in the fetus and infant and again at puberty. Despite the varying growth rates of different organ systems, there is an overall harmony of proportions. As an example, teeth are

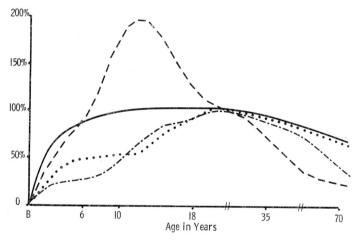

Growth and Degeneration Patterns of Systems

- − − Lymphoid System
- ——— Central Nervous System
- −·−·− Dentition
- • • • • General Body

Fig. 3. Graphic representation of the varying proportions (per cent) of the different organ systems in postnatal life. One hundred per cent represents the size of the organ systems in the mature young adult. (*Based on Scammon, R. E., 1930.*)

11

initiated and grow at the precise time that the jaws have reached a size ready to accommodate them.

The apparently scattered order of eruption of the teeth is another manifestation of the phenomenon of differing rates of growth. The various categories of teeth erupt at different times. The growth and development sequence is genetically determined and operates through the mechanism of inductors, metabolic modulators, neurotrophic and hormonal substances and interacting systems of contact stimulation and inhibition of contiguous tissues. Should these differential, but integrated, rates of development fail to maintain their normal determined 'pace', aberrations of total development will manifest themselves as malformations that may require clinical interception for correction.

Maturation is a counterpart of growth and indicates not only the attainment of adult size and proportions, but also the full adult constituents of tissues (e.g., mineralization) and the complete capability for performance of the organ's destined functions.

When the age of occurrence of maturational events is indicated (onset of ossification centres, fusion of sutures, eruption of teeth, etc.), it must be stressed that these manifestations of *biological age* of an individual need not coincide with *chronological age* and, in fact, they often differ from one another. When biological age is well in advance of chronological age, the individual is developing rapidly; when the reverse occurs, the individual exhibits a retarded rate of development.

While growth normally ceases at the end of adolescence, corresponding with the age of eruption of the third molar teeth (hence the popular connotation of 'wisdom teeth'), the facial bones, unlike the long bones, retain the potential for further appositional growth in adult life. Such post-adolescent growth may occur as a result of hypersecretion of somatotrophic hormone from a pituitary gland tumour, in the condition of acromegaly, characterized by an increase in the size of the bones of the face, hands and feet.

Early Embryonic Development

The development of the embryo may be conveniently divided into three main periods during the 280 days of its gestation (10 lunar months of 28 days each).* The *period of the ovum* extends from

---

*This duration of gestation is based upon the menstrual cycle of 28 days. Calculation from the last occurring menstruation is known as the 'menstrual age' of the embryo. This 'menstrual age' is most frequently used in obstetric practice, as it is based upon the last occurrence of an easily observed clinical symptom. As ovulation and subsequent fertilization occur approximately 14 days after the last menstruation, the true age of the embryo ('fertilization age') is two weeks less than the 'menstrual age'. Since they are more accurate, all ages referred to hereafter are 'fertilization ages', unless otherwise specified. To distinguish from postnatal ages, prenatal ages are indicated as being intra-uterine, abbreviated to i.u.

conception until the 7th or 8th day. The *embryonic period*, from the second through eighth weeks, may be subdivided into *presomite, somite*, and *postsomite* periods. The final *period of the fetus* encompasses the 3rd to 10th lunar months.

During the period of the ovum the cells of the zygote are undergoing rapid mitosis while it is travelling along the uterine tube to reach the uterus. By the end of this period, the migrating zygote, known at this time as the *blastocyst*, has implanted in the maternal uterine decidua.

The *presomite period* extends from the 8th to the 20th days of development, during which time the nutritional *fetal membranes* are established, and the *primary germ layers* are formed.

The *somite period* covers the 21st to 31st days of development. During this ten-day period, the basic patterns of the main systems and organs are established.

The *postsomite period*, from the 4th to 8th weeks, is characterized by rapid growth of the systems and organs established in the somite period, and by the formation of the main features of external body form.

During the *fetal period*, from the 3rd month until birth, there is little organogenesis or tissue differentiation, but there is rapid growth of the fetus.

1. *The Period of the Ovum*

During the period of the ovum, the cells of the zygote undergo rapid mitosis whereby the large cytoplasm:nucleus ratio of the original ovum is reduced in the resulting *blastomere* cells to the ratio found in general somatic cells. The increasingly numerous but smaller blastomeres do not increase the total size of the zygote until the end of the period of the ovum.

The solid cluster of cells (blastomeres) forming the *morula* that develops from the fertilized ovum (*Fig. 4*) accumulates fluid within its centre on the 4th day after conception to form a cyst-like structure termed the *blastocyst*. The outer ring of cells enclosing the fluid

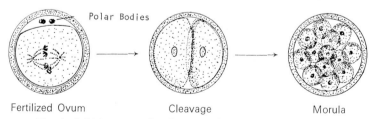

Fertilized Ovum   Cleavage   Morula

Fig. 4. Initial stages of embryogenesis, depicting cell division. Note that the morula, containing up to 16 cells, is no larger than the fertilized ovum.

13

forms the *trophoblast* that contains a cluster of cells known as the *inner cell mass* (*Fig. 5*A). At this stage, on the 7th day of development, the zygote, having travelled along the uterine tube, implants in the uterine wall by the process of nidation (*Fig. 5*B). The hitherto free-floating embryo's nutritional sources are thereby established by the formation of a *placenta*.

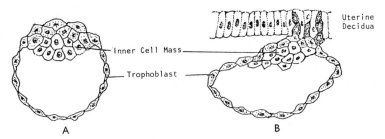

Uterine
Decidua

Inner Cell Mass

Trophoblast

A   B

Fig. 5. The blastocyst (**A**), developed from the morula, implants (**B**) into the decidual layer of the uterine wall.

2. The Embryonic Period

a. The Presomite Period.—Further development of the implanted zygote leads to the development of a number of extra-embryonic structures, termed the *fetal membranes*, and the development of the *embryo* itself. The fetal membranes are designed to protect the embryo and to serve its nutritional and waste disposal requirements. The main fetal membranes are the *chorion* and *amnion*; in the case of human development, combined later in the *umbilical cord* are the less important *yolk-sac* and *allantois* (*Figs. 10, 11*, pp. 17, 18).

The chorion develops from the blastocyst by the growth of villi into the surrounding maternal uterine decidua to tap the bloodsupply of the latter. The surface-directed villi eventually atrophy, while the basally-directed villi hypertrophy and combine with the uterine decidua basalis to form the *placenta* (*Fig. 6*A).

The amnion and yolk-sac develop within the inner cell mass as different sized sacs devoted to the protection, nutritional exchange, and waste elimination of the embryo. The two sacs arise by fluid accumulation between cells of the inner cell mass, separated by a bilaminar plate that will give rise to the embryo proper (*Fig. 6*B).

The two cell layers of the bilaminar plate or *germ disk* form two of the primary germ layers: the *ectoderm*, which forms the floor of the amniotic cavity, and the *endoderm*, which forms the roof of the yolk-sac (*Fig. 8*). Early demarcation, at the 14th day, of the anterior pole of the initially oval disk occurs by the appearance of an endo-

14

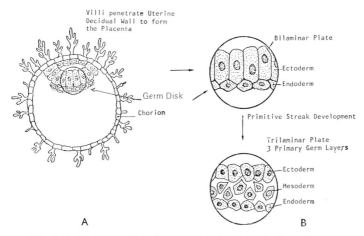

Fig. 6. A, The finger-like villi extending from the chorion adjacent to the inner cell mass form the fetal part of the placenta. B, Magnified sections of the germ disk depict its conversion from a 2-cell layered bilaminar plate to a 3-cell layered trilaminar plate.

dermal thickening, the *prechordal plate** in the future mid-cephalic region (*Figs. 7, 9*). The prechordal plate prefaces the development of the orofacial region since it later gives rise to the endodermal layer of the *oropharyngeal membrane*, the importance of which will be discussed later in the development of the mouth. The third primary germ layer, the *mesoderm*, makes its appearance at the beginning of the 3rd week as a result of ectodermal cell proliferation and differentiation in the caudal region of the germ disk. The resultant bulge in the disk is grooved craniocaudally, by which characteristic it is termed the *primitive streak* (*Fig. 9*). From the primitive streak the rapidly proliferating tissue known as *mesenchyme* forms the intra-embryonic mesoderm that migrates in all directions between the ectoderm and endoderm, except at the sites of the oropharyngeal membrane anteriorly and the *cloacal membrane* posteriorly (*Figs. 10, 11*). The appearance of the mesoderm converts the bilaminar germ disk into a trilaminar structure. The midline axis becomes defined by the formation of the *notochord* from the proliferation and differentiation of the cranial end of the primitive streak. The notochord terminates anteriorly at the prechordal plate (hence the latter's name) and marks the site of future pituitary gland development. The notochord serves as the axial skeleton of the embryo.

---

*The prechordal plate is believed to perform a head organizing function, and is postulated to give rise to cephalic mesenchyme concerned with extrinsic eye muscle development.

15

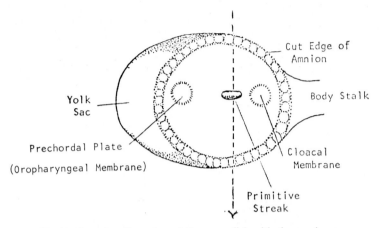

Fig. 7. Dorsal surface view of the germ disk with the amnion removed, depicting development of the primitive streak, and location
of the oropharyngeal and cloacal membranes. The interrupted line
is the plane of the coronal section of *Fig. 8.*

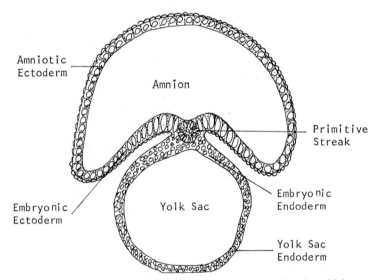

Fig. 8. Coronal section through the germ disk, showing the initial
fetal membranes, the amnion, and yolk-sac, above and below the
trilaminar germ disk. The primitive streak is the precursor of the
notochord, the central axis of the embryo.

16

The roof of the primitive gut (archenteron) induces formation of the neural plate in the overlying ectoderm (neural ectoderm) while the lateral mesoderm induces epidermal development (cutaneous ectoderm) (*Figs. 12, 13*).

The three primary germ layers serve as a basis for differentiating the tissues and organs that are largely derived from each of the

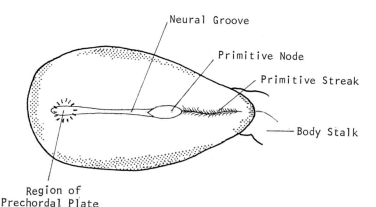

Fig. 9. Dorsal surface view of pear-shaped germ disk, with amnion cover removed, showing the location of the prechordal plate that presages future mouth development. The body stalk will form the umbilical cord connecting the embryo to the placenta.

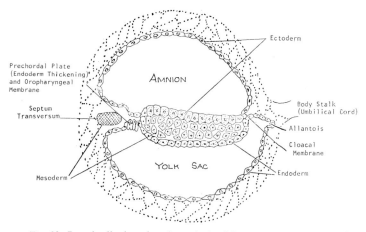

Fig. 10. Longitudinal section through the differentiating germ disk, with ectoderm-endoderm contact maintained at the prechordal plate (precursor of the orofacial region) and at the cloacal membrane (precursor of the uroanal region). The mesoderm of the septum transversum contributes to the liver and diaphragm.

17

layers. From the ectoderm the cutaneous and neural systems develop. The cutaneous structures include the skin and its appendages, the oral mucous membrane, and the enamel of teeth. The neural structures include the central and peripheral nervous systems. The mesoderm gives rise to the cardiovascular system (heart and blood-vessels), the locomotor system (bones and muscles), the connective tissues, and the pulp, dentine, periodontal ligament, and cementum of teeth. The endoderm develops into the lining epithelium of the alimentary canal between the pharynx and the anus, and the secretory cells of the liver and pancreas, as well as the lining epithelium of the respiratory system.

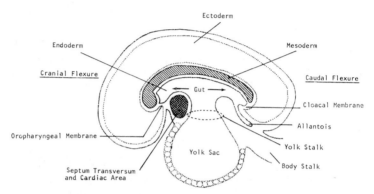

Fig. 11. Longitudinal section through the presomite embryo depicting the closing off of the yolk-sac from the gut, at the yolk stalk, and the cranial and caudal boundaries of the gut at the oropharyngeal and cloacal membranes.

Development of the ectoderm into its cutaneous and neural portions occurs by the infolding of the *neural plate* ectoderm along the midline forming the *neural folds* that fuse to form the *neural tube* that submerges beneath the superficial covering cutaneous ectoderm (*Figs. 13, 14*). Arising from the margins of the crests of the neural folds are *neural crest cells* first appearing in 7–14 somite stage embryos. These neural crest cells develop as a result of interactions between the neuralizing and epidermalizing influences on ectoderm, accounting for the crestal location where the neuralizing and epidermalizing zones meet. These cells form a separate transitory tissue akin to the primary germ cell types. Neural crest cells, although of ectodermal origin, exhibit most of the properties associated with mesenchyme; as a result the tissue they form is termed *ectomesenchyme*. Ectomesenchyme possesses great migratory propensities, appearing to follow the natural cleavage planes between

18

mesoderm, ectoderm and endoderm. In migrating from their site of formation, neural crest cells possess an inherent migratory pattern that may be influenced by environmental factors along routes that form as cell-free pathways filled with a filamentous mesh. The migrating neural crest cells are bipolar, their elongated form being orientated in the direction of migration. The mechanism of crest cell movement is unknown, although they exhibit filopodia (microspikes) that contact adjacent cells and structures. Migrating neural crest cells, upon reaching their destinations, undergo cyto-differentiation into a wide variety of diverse cell types that are in

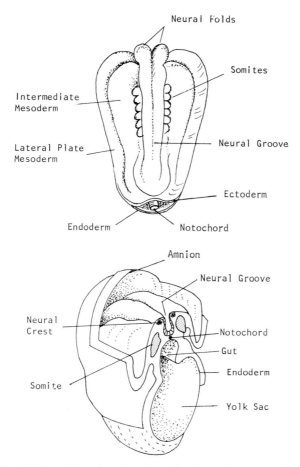

Fig. 12. Upper. Dorsal surface view of early somite stage embryo depicting neural groove formation. *Lower,* Sectioned view of early somite stage embryo.

19

part specified by local environmental influences. Specific sites for the arrest of migrating crest cells are present in the embryo. Besides forming chromaffin tissue (adrenal medulla, etc.), ectomesenchyme contributes to a number of diverse structures, both at the site of the tissue's dorsolateral origin and in remote regions of the body.

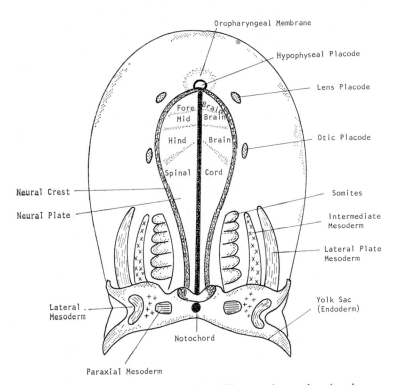

Fig. 13. Composite 'fate map' of the different regions and sectioned view of the cranial end of an early somite period embryo.

Neural crest cell clusters adjacent to the neural tube form the ganglia of the autonomic nervous system and of sensory nerves, both spinal and cranial—the facial, glossopharyngeal and vagus ganglia. Part of the trigeminal ganglion (the other part is derived from cranial placodes) and the carotid body are of neural crest origin. The neural crest cells migrate to form Schwann cells surrounding nerve-fibres and pigment cells of epidermis (melanocytes). Crest cells contribute to the leptomeninges (arachnoid and pia mater) and the scleral and choroid optic coats. They further give rise to the

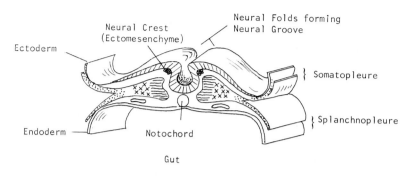

Paraxial Mesoderm

Intermediate Mesoderm

Lateral Mesoderm

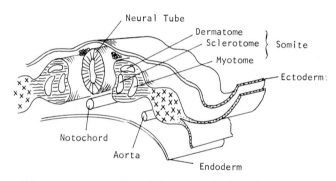

Fig. 14. Schematic representation of late presomite (*above*) and somite (*below*) stages of development, depicting neural tube formation and mesoderm differentiation.

cartilages of the branchial arches★ and the osteoblasts that form intramembranous skull bones. Neural crest cells contribute to the facial processes, and are the precursors of the odontoblast cells of the dental pulp that will subsequently form the dentine of teeth.†

  b. The Somite Period.—The basic tissue types having developed during the first 21 days, the next 10 days of development are

---

★The environment of the branchial arches is rich in cartilage-promoting influences —chondroitin sulphate, chondro-mucoprotein etc.

†It has been postulated that this mechanism of remotely neural origin of dentine might account for its exquisite sensitivity. This hypothesis presumes dentine to be deviously derived from neural tissue.

21

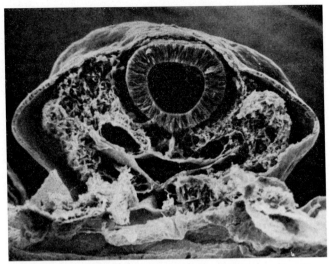

Fig. 15. Scanning electron micrograph of a Hamburger–Hamilton Stage 10 chick embryo sectioned immediately posterior to the optic vesicle, showing the neural tube, the mesodermal mass of cells and the surface ectoderm which is separated from the mesoderm by a 'cell free space' through which cranial neural crest cells migrate. (×150.) (*By courtesy of A. J. Steffek and D. K. Mujwid, American Dental Association, Research Institute, Health Foundation, Chicago.*)

characterized by foldings and structuring, as well as by differentiation of the basic tissues that convert the flat embryonic disk into a tubular body (*Figs. 14, 16*). The first of these changes (21 days) is the folding of the neural plate, from which the brain and spinal cord develop. Next, the mesoderm develops into three aggregations—the lateral plate, intermediate, and paraxial mesoderm, each with a different fate. The lateral plate mesoderm contributes to the walls of the embryonic coelom from which the pleural, pericardial, and peritoneal cavities develop. The intermediate mesoderm contributes to the formation of the gonad, kidney, and adrenal cortex. The paraxial mesoderm, alongside the notochord, divides into a series of segmental blocks, termed *somites*, whose prominence characterizes this period (21st to 31st days) of embryonic development (*Fig. 17*). The 42–44 paired somites appear sequentially in a craniocaudal direction and set the pattern for the regions of the body by their being identified as 4 occipital, 8 cervical, 12 thoracic, 5 lumbar, 5 sacral, and 8–10 coccygeal somites (*Fig. 17*).

Each somite differentiates into three parts whose fates are implied in their names. The ventromedial part is designated the *sclerotome**;

---

*Proteoglycans (procollagen) and collagen secreted by the notochord induce the conversion of somite sclerotomal cells into cartilage.

EARLY EMBRYONIC DEVELOPMENT

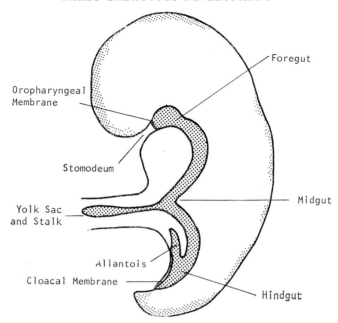

Fig. 16. Schematic longitudinal section through a somite period embryo depicting the subdivisions of the gut.

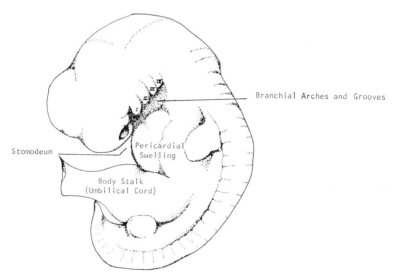

Fig. 17. Surface view of late somite period embryo (31 days) showing conspicuous somites along the back and the development of the branchial arches and limb buds.

23

it contributes to the vertebral column and accounts for its segmental nature, except in the occipital region, where fusion occurs to form the occipital skull-bone. The lateral aspect of the somite is termed the *dermatome*, and gives rise to the dermis of the skin. The intermediate portion, the *myotome*, differentiates into muscles of the trunk and limbs and may contribute to some of the muscles of the orofacial region.

The somite period is characterized by the establishment of most of the organ systems of the embryo. The cardiovascular, alimentary, respiratory, genito-urinary, and nervous systems are established and the primordia of the eye and the internal ear appear during this period. The embryonic disk develops lateral and head and tail folds, facilitating the enclosure of the endodermal germ layer from the yolk-sac, thereby laying the basis for the tubular intestine. The part of the yolk-sac endoderm incorporated into the cranial end of the embryo is termed the *foregut*, the anterior boundary of which is closed off by the oropharyngeal membrane. Similarly, the part of the yolk-sac incorporated into the caudal end of the embryo is termed the *hindgut*, bounded ventrally by the cloacal membrane. The intervening portion of the alimentary canal is called the *midgut*, which remains in communication with the yolk-sac through the *yolk stalk* (*Fig. 16*). The gut is initially sealed off at both ends, and is only converted into a canal by the later breakdown of the oropharyngeal and cloacal membranes.

The foregut endoderm later gives rise to the *laryngotracheal diverticulum* from which the bronchi and lungs develop. Other endodermal outgrowths from the foregut are the *hepatic* and *pancreatic diverticula*, giving rise to the secretory elements of the liver and pancreas. The foregut itself develops into the pharynx and its important *pharyngeal pouches*, the oesophagus, stomach, and first part of the duodenum. The midgut forms the rest of the duodenum, the entire small intestine, and the ascending and transverse colon of the large intestine. The hindgut forms the descending colon and the terminal parts of the alimentary canal.

The external appearance of the late somite embryo presents a prominent brain forming a predominant portion of the early head, whose 'face' and 'neck', formed by branchial arches, is strongly flexed over a precocious heart. The eyes, nose, and ears are demarcated by placodes, while ventrolateral swellings indicate the beginnings of the limb buds. The lower belly wall protrudes conspicuously in its connexions with the placenta through the body stalk and a prominent tail terminates the caudal end of the embryo (*Figs. 17, 18*).

The extremely complex and very rapid basic organogenesis taking place during the 10-day somite period makes the embryo exceedingly susceptible to environmental disturbances that may produce

24

permanent developmental derangements. Maternal illnesses, particularly of viral origin, and drug therapy during the first trimester of pregnancy, which includes the somite period of development, are well known in obstetric practice to be the cause of congenital deformities of the fetus.

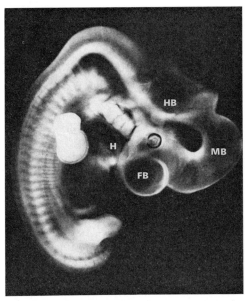

Fig. 18. Lateral view of a human embryo in the late somite period (early in the 5th week). Note the forebrain (FB), containing the prominent eye, the midbrain (MB) and hindbrain (HB). The primitive face is flexed in contact with the prominent heart (H). The somites are evident as dorsal segments continuing into a tail. The upper and lower limb buds are seen as prominent paddle-shaped projections. (*By courtesy of Professor Dr E. Blechschmidt.*)

c. The Postsomite Period.—The predominance of the segmental somites as an external feature of the early embryo fades during the 6th week i.u.* The head dominates much of the development of this period. Facial features become recognizable, when the ears, eyes, and nose assume a 'human' form, and the neck becomes defined by its elongation and the sheathing of the branchial arches. The paddle-shaped limb buds of the early part of the period expand and differentiate into their divisions down to the first demarcation of their digits. The earliest muscular movements are first manifest at this time. The body stalk of the previous periods condenses into a

---

*i.u. = intra-uterine.

definitive umbilical cord as it becomes less conspicuous on the belly wall. The thoracic region swells enormously, as the heart, which becomes very prominent in the somite period, is joined by the rapidly growing liver, whose size dominates the early abdominal organs. The long tail of the beginning of the embryonic period regresses as the growing buttocks aid in its concealment. The embryo at the end of this period is now termed a 'fetus'.

3. The Fetal Period

The main organs and systems having developed during the somite and embryonic periods, the last 6 months of fetal life are devoted to very rapid growth and re-proportioning of body components, with little further organogenesis or tissue differentiation. The precocious growth and development of the head in the embryonic period is not maintained in the fetal period, with the result that the body develops relatively more rapidly. Accordingly, the proportions of the head are reduced from about one-half of the entire body length at the beginning of the fetal period to about one-third at the 5th month, and to about one-fourth at birth. At 4 months i.u. the face assumes a human appearance as the laterally directed eyes move to the front of the face and the ears rise from their original mandibulocervical site to eye-level. The limbs grow rapidly, although disproportionately, the lower limbs lagging in comparison with the upper. Ossification centres make their appearance in most of the bones during this period. The sex of the fetus can be observed externally by the 3rd month, and the wrinkled skin acquires a covering of downy hairs ('lanugo') by the 5th month. During this month, fetal movements are first felt by the mother. The sebaceous glands of the skin become very active just prior to birth (7th and 8th months), covering the fetus with their fatty secretions, termed the 'vernix caseosa' (*vernix*, varnish; *caseosa*, cheesy). In the last two months of fetal life, fat deposits subcutaneously to fill out the wrinkled skin, and nearly half the ultimate birth-weight is added in this time.

Despite the rapid growth of the postcranial portions of the body during the fetal period, the head still has the largest circumference of all the parts of the body at birth. The passage of the head through the birth canal has to be accommodated by its compression. The birth compression of the cranium presents the danger of distortion; this normally rectifies itself postnatally, but may persist as a source of perverted mandibulofacial development.

SELECTED BIBLIOGRAPHY

Arey, L. B. (1965), *Developmental Anatomy*, 7th ed. Philadelphia: Saunders.

BAER, M. (1973), *Growth and Maturation.* Cambridge, Mass.: Howard A. Doyle.

BENIRSHKE, K., LOWRY, R. B., OPITZ, J. M., SCHWARZACHER, H. G., and SPRANGER, J. W. (1979), 'Developmental Terms—Some Proposals', *Am. J. Med. Gen.*, **3**, 297.

BLECHSCHMIDT, E. (1977), *The Beginnings of Human Life*, New York: Springer-Verlag.

— —and GASSER, R. F. (1978), *Biokinetics and Biodynamics of Human Differentiation.* Springfield, Ill.: Thomas.

BRACHET, J. (1974), *Introduction to Molecular Embryology.* London: English Universities Press.

FALKNER, F. (Ed.) (1966), *Human Development.* Philadelphia: Saunders.

FITZGERALD, M. J. T. (1978), *Human Embryology: a Regional Approach.* Hagerstown, MD.: Harper & Row.

GARROD, D. R. (1978), *Specificity of Embryological Interactions.* London: Chapman & Hall.

HAM, R. G., and VEOMETT, M. J. (1979), *Mechanisms of Development.* St. Louis: Mosby.

HAMILTON, W. J., and MOSSMAN, H. W. (1972), *Human Embryology*, 4th ed. Cambridge: Heffer.

MCNAMARA, J. A., JUN. (Ed.) 1975, *Control Mechanisms in Craniofacial Growth.* Monograph No. 3, Craniofacial Growth Series, Center for Human Growth and Development. Ann Arbor: University of Michigan.

MOORE, K. (1977), *The Developing Human*, 2nd ed. Philadelphia: Saunders.

MOSS, M. L. (1969), 'Phylogeny and Comparative Anatomy of Oral Ectodermal–ectomesenchymal Inductive Interactions', *J. dent. Res.*, **48**, 732.

NISHIMURA, H., SEMBA, R., TANIMURA, T., and TANKA, O. (1977), *Prenatal Development of the Human with Special Reference to Craniofacial Structures: An Atlas.* DHEW Publication No. (NIH) 77–946. Washington: U.S. Government Printing Office.

O'RAHILLY, R. (1973), *Developmental Stages in Human Embryos.* Publication 631, Carnegie Institution of Washington, D.C.

PARKE, W. W. (1975). *Photographic Atlas of Fetal Anatomy.* Baltimore: University Park Press.

PATTEN, B. M., and CARLSON, B. M. (1974), *Foundations of Embryology*, 3rd ed. New York: McGraw-Hill.

SCAMMON, R. E. (1930), 'The Measurement of the Body in Childhood', in *The Measurement of Man* (Ed. HARRIS, J. A.), p. 50. Minneapolis: University of Minnesota Press.

SLAVKIN, H. (1979), *Developmental Craniofacial Biology.* Philadelphia: Lea & Febiger.

STEWART, R. E., and PRESSCOTT, G. H. (1976), *Oral Facial Genetics.* St. Louis: Mosby.

VALDES-DAPENA, M. A. (1979), *Histology of the Fetus and Newborn.* Philadelphia: Saunders.

CHAPTER 3

EARLY OROFACIAL DEVELOPMENT

ORAL development in the embryo is demarcated extremely early in life by the appearance of the *prechordal plate* in the bilaminar germ disk on the 14th day of development, even prior to the appearance of the mesodermal germ layer. The endodermal thickening of the prechordal plate designates the cranial pole of the oval embryonic disk, and later contributes to the *oropharyngeal membrane*. This tenuous and temporary bilaminar membrane serves as the site of junction of the ectoderm that forms the mucosa of the mouth and the endoderm that forms the mucosa of the pharynx, which is the most cranial part of the foregut. The oropharyngeal membrane is one of two sites of contiguity between ectoderm and endoderm, where mesoderm fails to intervene between the two primary germ layers; the other site is the *cloacal membrane* at the terminal end of the hind gut. The oropharyngeal membrane also demarcates the site of a shallow depression, the *stomodeum*, the primitive mouth that forms the topographical centre of the developing face.

Rapid orofacial development is characteristic of the advanced development of the cranial portion of the embryo when compared

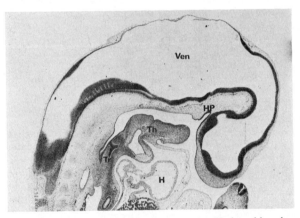

Fig. 19. Sagittal section of head region of a 32-day-old embryo. The ventricles (Ven) occupy a large proportion of the brain. The hypophyseal pouch (HP) extends up from the stomodeum that is bordered below by the heart (H). The thyroid gland (Th) is seen budding from the foramen caecum in the tongue via the thyroglossal duct. The trachea (Tr) is budding from the primitive oseophagus. (×22.) (*By courtesy of Professor H. Nishimura.*)

with its caudal portion. The differential rates of growth result in a pear-shaped embryonic disk, with the head region forming the expanded portion of the pear (*see Fig. 9*, p. 17). Further, the three germ layers in the cranial part of the embryo begin their specific development by the middle of the 3rd week, while the separation of the germ layers still continues in the caudal portion up to the end of the 4th week. The precocious development of the cranial end of the embryo results in the head constituting nearly one-half of the total body size during the postsomite embryonic period (4th to 8th weeks). Subsequent postcranial development results in the head forming one-quarter the body length at birth and being only 6–8 per cent of the body in adulthood.

In the early part of the somite stage (21st to 31st days) of development, the 3 mm. long embryo develops at its cranial end five mesenchymal elevations or 'processes' that correspond to centres of growth in the underlying mesenchyme and are caused by neural crest ectomesenchymal migration (*Fig. 19*). The migrating mesenchyme insinuating between the outer ectoderm and inner endoderm creates bulges that 'heap up' into facial elevations. The difference between a 'hill' and a 'valley' or between a prominence and a groove is dependent upon the amount of mesenchyme between the two epithelial layers. The blending of the facial prominences is merely the filling in of the valleys or grooves by migrating mesenchyme. Inadequate mesenchymal migration* results in persistence of the grooves with subsequent epithelial breakdown and consequent cleft formation.

Neural crest tissue migrates forward around the developing brain from its initial dorsal location, losing contact with the neural tube, except at the points of exit of the cranial nerves (*Fig. 20*). At this time the forebrain develops evaginations, the *optic vesicles*, that are the precursors of the eyes, and that induce conspicuous *lens placodes* in the overlying ectoderm. Placodes† are areas of thick ectoderm of the embryonic head that differentiate into sense organs (sight, smell and hearing) and form elements of the peripheral nervous system (sensory ganglia of the trigeminal, facial, glossopharyngeal and vagus nerves). Where the migrating sheet of neural crest cells encounters the eye, it splits into anterior and posterior

---

*It appears that accumulating detrimental genetic and/or environmental influences may progressively reduce the amount of facial ectomesenchyme, and if reduced below a certain threshold, facial clefts will result.

†Placodes first become visible as separate areas of thick ectoderm because the surrounding ectoderm grows thinner. Placodes thus do not initially thicken, but maintain the initial ectodermal thickness. Actual thickening of the placodes occurs later. The major portion of ectoderm thins to cover rapidly expanding surfaces, and by the migration of ectodermal mesenchyme (neural crest) away from the surface.

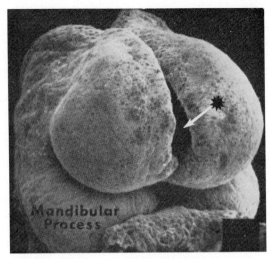

Fig. 20. Scanning electron photomicrograph of the 'face' of an 8¼-day-old hamster embryo. The ★ marks the anterior opening of the neural tube. No maxillary processes have yet formed, and the mandibular arches on either side of the stomodeum have not yet met in the midline (×118.) (*By courtesy of Waterman, R. E., and Meller, S. M., 1973*, 'Nasal Pit Formation in the Hamster', *Dev. Biol.*, **34**, 255. *By kind permission of Academic Press Inc.*)

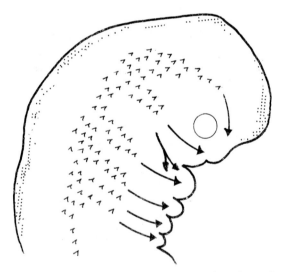

Fig. 21. Schematic representation of the migration of neural crest tissue (arrows) from the site of its dorsal origin into the facial and branchial regions.

streams. The anterior stream is responsible for forming the mesenchyme of the *frontonasal process*, while the posterior stream enters
the *branchial arches* to contribute to their mesenchyme. At the end
of neural crest migration, the ectomesenchyme differentiates into
several possible tissues that is determined by the environment in
which it terminates (*see* p. 20). The swellings of the embryonic *facial
processes* result from the proliferation of their contained mesenchyme, from which the facial skeletal and connective tissues will
develop. The ectodermal grooves or furrows that lie between these
growth centres demarcate the facial processes. These surround a
central depression forming the stomodeum. The five prominences
that constitute the initial features of the face are a single central
most cranially located *frontonasal process* and the two bilaterally
located *maxillary processes* and *mandibular arches*, both derived
from the first of the *branchial arches*, that are part of the branchial
arch system (p. 51). The masses or processes grow differentially,
and by obliterating the ectodermal grooves between them provide
an eventually even contour to the features of the face. As a result
of a flexure (the cranial flexure) developing in the future mandibulo-
cervical region, the primitive face is bent over the enormous heart
region during its early development (*see Figs. 11* and *17*, pp. 18 and
23 and *Fig. 19*, p. 28).

In the region of the dorsal end of the first branchial groove,
between the first and second branchial arches and overlying the

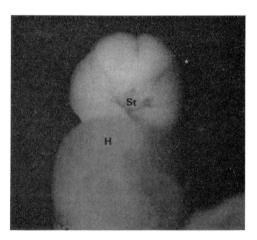

Fig. 22. Face of a 24-day-old embryo. The oropharyngeal membrane lines the stomodeum (St). The forebrain above the stomodeum is partially subdivided into telencephalic hemispheres. Note
the very prominent heart (H). (×50.) (*By courtesy of Professor H.
Nishimura.*)

CRANIOFACIAL EMBRYOLOGY

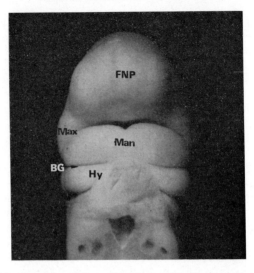

Fig. 23. Face of a 28-day-old embryo. The frontonasal process
(FNP), maxillary process (Max) and mandibular process (Man.)
border the stomodeum. The first branchial groove (B.G.) demarcates the first branchial arch from the second branchial (hyoid-Hy)
arch. The oropharyngeal membrane has just disintegrated. ($\times$32.)
(*By courtesy of Professor H. Nishimura.*)

hindbrain there develops an epithelial thickening, the *otic placode*,
that is a precursor of the inner ear (p. 181). While the placode
rapidly sinks beneath the surface as the *otic vesicle*, it demarcates the
location of the future external ear (*see* p. 180).

The wide frontonasal process intervenes between the laterally
placed developing eyes, and will contribute to the forehead and nose.
The olfactory portion of the latter organ develops from *nasal
(olfactory) placodes* that form from specialized epithelial thickenings
at the inferolateral corners of the frontonasal process (*Figs. 22, 23*).
The growth of the horseshoe-shaped *medial* and *lateral nasal processes* surrounding each of the sinking nasal placodes during the 5th
week creates deepening *nasal pits* that form the anterior nares (*Figs.
24, 25, 26*). The posterior aspect of each nasal pit is initially separated
from the oral cavity by the *oronasal (bucconasal) membrane* that
disintegrates by the end of the 5th week. Disintegration of the
oronasal membrane creates posterior openings of the nasal pits—
the *choanae* opening into the roof of the primitive oral cavity.

The elevation of the lateral nasal processes creates the alae of
the nose. The medial tip of the maxillary process extends medially
to contact the inferolateral side of the medial nasal process, but is

32

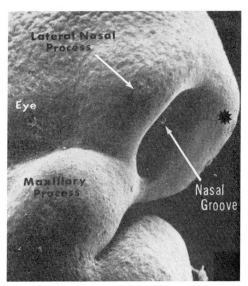

Fig. 24. Scanning electron photomicrograph of the lateral aspect of a 9¼-day-old hamster embryo. The ★ demarcates the medial nasal process, that becomes continuous inferiorly with the maxillary process. The region of the developing eye is identified. (×68.) (*By courtesy of Waterman, R. E., and Meller, S. M., 1973,* 'Nasal Pit Formation in the Hamster', *Dev. Biol.,* **34**, 255. *By kind permission of Academic Press Inc.*)

initially separated by an epithelial *nasal fin*★ that soon degenerates, allowing maxillary mesenchyme to merge with medial nasal mesenchyme. The medial nasal processes approach each other to form a single *globular process* that forms the tip of the nose, the columella, the philtrum† and labial tuberculum of the upper lip (the prolabium)‡ the frenulum and the entire primary palate (*Fig. 30*). This median palatal primordium will later contain the upper incisor teeth and is continuous above with the most ventral portion of the nasal septum.

The *nasal septum* develops from the roof of the stomodeum as a

---

★Persistence of the nasal fin has been postulated to be a cause of cleft lip and anterior cleft palate by preventing merging of maxillary and medial nasal process mesenchyme.

†The philtrum forms between the 3rd and 4th month i.u. as a vertical median groove of the upper lip. The paramedian eminences, resulting from mesenchymal connective tissue migrating tardily between the skin and orbicularis oris muscle, arise at the sites of the much earlier merging of maxillary and globular processes, but appear to be developmentally dissociated from these 'junctions'.

‡The embryological origins of the definitive upper lip are disputed. Some embryologists maintain that the globular process is overgrown by the two maxillary processes in normal development, but clefts formed in abnormal development refute this view.

midsagittal projection of the cartilage floor of the forebrain. The cartilage septum divides the nasal cavity into left and right nasal fossae. Invasion of ectoderm into the median nasal septum from both nasal fossae creates the vestigial *vomeronasal organ* * (*Fig. 62*). Similar ectodermal invasions into the lateral walls of the fossae form the *superior, middle* and *inferior nasal meatus*, in increasing order of size, that will separate swellings forming the *superior, middle* and *inferior nasal conchae*. The conchae are initially cartilaginous extensions of the nasal capsule projecting from the lateral walls of each nasal fossa. Later ossification of the cartilages forms the bony conchae.

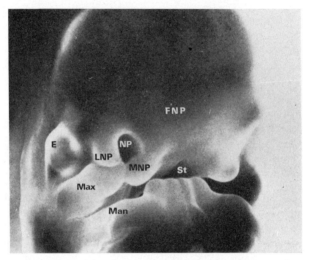

Fig. 25. Face of a late somite period (30–32 days) human embryo. The frontonasal process (FNP) projects the medial nasal (MNP) and lateral nasal process (LNP) on each side, surrounding the nasal placode (NP). The eye (E) is seen in its lateral position. The maxillary process (Max) forms the superolateral boundary of the stomodeum (St) and the mandibular process forms the lower boundary. (*By courtesy of Professor Dr E. Blechschmidt.*)

The maxillary growth centres or processes of each side, that will form the lateral part of the lip, cheek and maxilla, merge with the frontonasal process by the smoothing out of their separating furrows to provide continuity of the upper lip and cheek regions.

---

*The vomeronasal organ (of Jacobson) is a rudimentary olfactory sac that invaginates both sides of the nasal septum between the 6th and 8th weeks i.u. The sac closes to form a blind pouch at the 20th week, reaching its fullest development at the 5th month i.u. Thereafter it diminishes and usually disappears, but may persist in the adult.

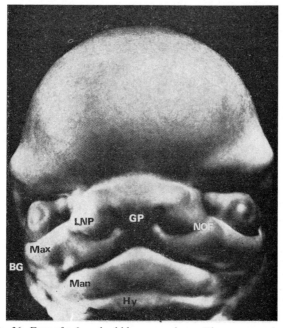

Fig. 26. Face of a 6-week-old human embryo. The eyes are migrating medially. The globular process (GP) has melded with the maxillary processes (Max) to form the upper lip. The lateral nasal process (LNP) is demarcated from the maxillary process by the naso-optic furrow (NOF), the precursor of the nasolacrimal duct. The first branchial groove (BG), the precursor of the external acoustic meatus, is located between the mandibular branchial arch (Mand) and the second branchial (hyoid) arch (Hy). (*By courtesy of Professor Dr E. Blechschmidt.*)

Some slight evidence of the diverse origins of the upper lip is provided by the 'Cupid's bow' outline ⌣⌣ of its upper margin, the central tuberculum being derived from the globular process and the lateral aspects from the maxillary processes. The two mandibular growth centres or processes merge in the midline by the filling in of their separate furrow* to provide continuity to the lower jaw and lip.

At the boundary line between the lateral nasal process and the maxillary process there develops a trough-like epithelial groove—

---

*The epithelium is pushed out from between the elevations, and no epithelial resorption occurs. Retardation of growth in the region of the furrow between merging processes accounts for clefts and inclusion cysts. Evidence suggests that the embryological facial furrows may influence the local spread of facial cancer. Epithelial tumour spread seems to be initially contained within the boundaries of the embryological processes. Tumours arising over furrow sites (boundaries) tend to invade deeply before spreading superficially.

35

the *naso-optic furrow* connecting the conjunctival lacrimal sac of the eye with the lateral wall of the nose (*Fig. 28*). The epithelial groove fuses into a canal to form the nasolacrimal duct that later drains tear fluid of the eye into the nose. Migration of the eyes from their lateral location towards the midline takes place as a result of relative narrowing of the intervening frontonasal process and expansion of the lateral aspects of the head (*Fig. 29*).

The primitive stomodeum outlined by the merging maxillary and mandibular processes extends from the developing floor of the mouth inferiorly to the chondrocranium superiorly. The stomodeum forms a shallow depression, limited in its depth by the oropharyngeal membrane. The characteristically deep oral cavity is formed by the forward growth of the processes surrounding the stomodeum. The stomodeum becomes established as an oronasopharyngeal chamber and entrance to the gut by the disintegration of the dividing oropharyngeal membrane at the 28th day, thereby providing continuity of passage between the mouth and the pharynx.* Division of the stomodeal chamber into separate oral and nasal cavities is first occasioned by the frontonasal and globular processes developing vertical and horizontal extensions into the chamber, forming the thick primitive *nasal septum* and *primary palate* respectively (*Fig. 30*). Inwardly directed processes—the *lateral palatal shelves*—develop from the maxillary processes bounding the stomodeum during the 6th week i.u., at which time the tongue is growing extremely rapidly, swelling up from the branchial arches (*Fig. 32*). The combination of a relatively small stomodeum having to accommodate a rapidly enlarging tongue during the 7th week i.u. results in the tongue completely filling the oronasal cavity (*Fig. 33*). The continued growth of the lateral palatal shelves during this time results in them being forced down into the only available space on either side of the root of the tongue. Development during the 8th week i.u. results in enlargement of the stomodeal chamber, enabling the tongue to drop into the lower part of the cavity, and freeing the vertical palatal shelves (*Figs. 34, 35*). The unencumbered palatal shelves now swing or possibly flow in a wave-like fashion into an horizontal plane, and establish contact with each other in the midline, with the primary palate anteriorly, and with the lower portion of the nasal septum (*Fig. 36*). Beginning about one-third of the way from

---

*While the oropharyngeal membrane demarcates the junction of ectoderm and endoderm in the embryo, this line of division is very difficult to trace subsequently due to the extensive changes occurring in oropharyngeal development. Since the hypophysis originates from Rathke's pouch anterior to the oropharyngeal membrane, a measure of the depth of oral growth is provided by its adult location. The presumed site of the original oropharyngeal membrane in the adult is an imaginary vertical plane from the posterior border of the body of the sphenoid bone through the tonsillar region of the fauces.

the front, the free edges of the lateral shelves meet, and the intervening epithelium breaks down, allowing the processes to fuse, proceeding both anteriorly and posteriorly. Fusion of the two processes starts in the 8th week and is usually completed by the 12th week i.u. Fusion also occurs with the nasal septum except posteriorly, where the soft palate and uvula remain unattached.

In the region of the future soft palate and uvula, a merging of invading mesenchyme (*see* p. 117) occurs across the midline junction. No ossification takes place in this region. The extraterritorial tissue invasion from the first, third and fourth branchial arches into the soft palate and faucial regions of the oropharynx accounts for the complicated innervation of this area in the adult.

Meanwhile, the lower free edge of the nasal septum has grown down to meet and fuse with the upper surfaces of the fusing palatal processes, thereby dividing the stomodeum into an oral cavity and two nasal fossae (*Fig. 36*). Development of the nasal capsules of the chondrocranium (*see* p. 89) later provides the cartilaginous element of the thinned definitive nasal septum. Separate ossification centres in the three palatal elements (*see* p. 116) provide the basis for the bony hard palate.

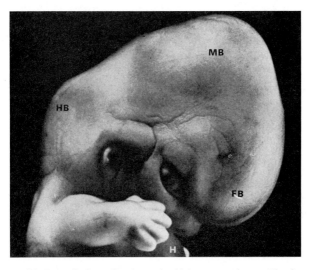

Fig. 27. Lateral view of a 6½-week-old human embryo. The face is strongly flexed over the prominent heart (H). Note the location of the forebrain (FB), midbrain (MB) and hindbrain (HB) and the first branchial groove forming the external acoustic meatus. The fingers are differentiating out of the hand paddle. Note the absence of eyelids and the prominent lens vesicle in the centre of the optic cup. (*By courtesy of Professor Dr E. Blechschmidt.*)

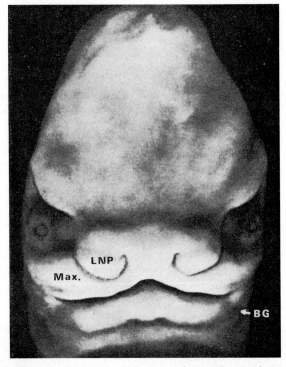

Fig. 28. Face of a 7-week-old human embryo. The nose is gradually projecting as the eyes migrate medially and the branchial groove (BG) rises on the side of the face. The naso-optic furrow is submerging between the lateral nasal process (LNP) and the maxillary process (Max). The upper lip is cupid-bow shaped. (*By courtesy of Professor Dr E. Blechschmidt.*)

Further development of the palate is dealt with in the chapter on the palate (p. 114).

The external opening of the stomodeum forms an abnormally wide mouth in the early stages of facial development. Reduction of the mouth orifice to normal proportions occurs by the filling in of the furrow between the maxillary and mandibular processes to a demarcated point, forming the corner of the mouth.

Within the primitive stomodeum, immediately ventral to the oropharyngeal membrane, there develops, as a result of a mesen-chymal-neural inductive process,* a deep fold or diverticulum of

---

*The prechordal plate is believed to be implicated in the early induction of the hypophyseal pouch. A remnant of the stomodeal diverticulum may occasionally be seen as a cleft in the fully formed adenohypophysis.

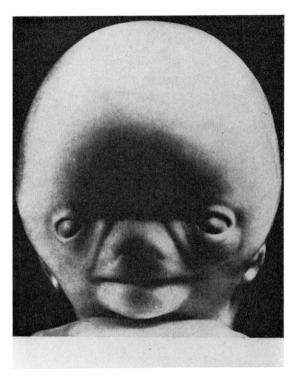

Fig. 29. Face of a 7-week-old human embryo. The relatively large forehead dominates the face. Eyelids are beginning to form above and below the migrating eyes. The mouth opening is reducing in size. (*By courtesy of Professor Dr E. Blechschmidt.*)

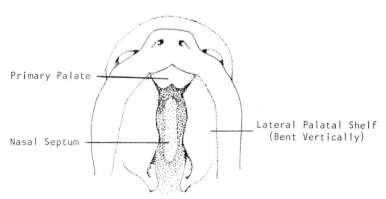

Fig. 30. View of the three primordia of the palate in the 7½-week-old embryo.

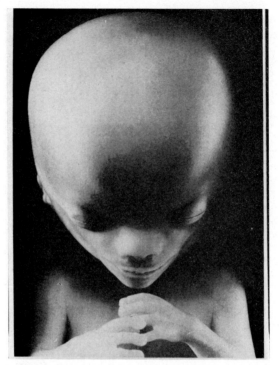

Fig. 31. Face of a 3-month-old fetus. The eyelids have completely formed and closed over the eyes. Medial migration of the eyes will narrow the interocular distance. Precocious brain development dominates the size of the head at this age.

Ossification has commenced to form the craniofacial skeleton. (*By courtesy of Professor Dr E. Blechschmidt.*)

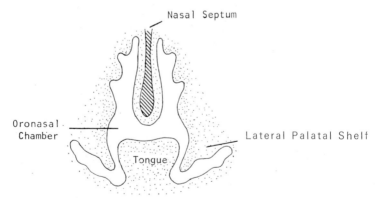

Fig. 32. Schematic coronal cross-section of stomodeal chamber in 7-week-old embryo, showing 'vertical' lateral palatal shelves.

the ectoderm in the roof of the primitive oral cavity. This diverticulum, known as the *hypophyseal pouch* or *Rathke's pouch*, gives rise to the anterior lobe of the pituitary gland (adenohypophysis) (*see Fig. 37*, p. 43). There is an ectodermal field in the stomodeum that is induced to form the hypophyseal pouch by the underlying

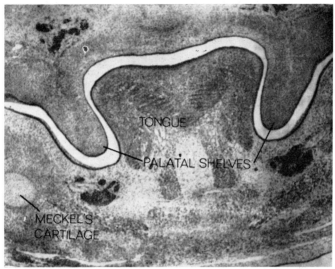

Fig. 33. Photomicrograph of coronal section of the stomodeum of a pig embryo, showing the tongue filling the oropharyngeal chamber, and the obliquely directed palatal shelves on either side of the tongue. (×40.)

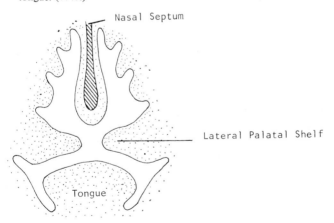

Fig. 34. Schematic coronal section of the stomodeal chamber of an 8-week-old human embryo, showing horizontal lateral palatal shelves.

41

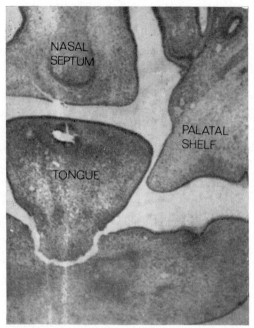

Fig. 35. Photomicrograph of coronal section of the stomodeum of a pig embryo showing the beginning of lateral palatal shelf elevation. (×40.)

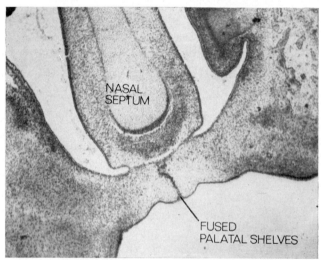

Fig. 36. Photomicrograph of coronal section of the oronasal region of a 10-week fetus, showing fusion of the lateral palatal shelves with each other, and with the nasal septum. (×40.)

42

prechordal mesenchyme. The hypophyseal pouch extends dorsally immediately anterior to the notochord through the ectomeningeal mesenchyme that will form the future postsphenoid (cranial base) bone towards the diencephalon of the forebrain. The extended hypophyseal pouch forms a duct and a terminal cord of initially stomodeal ectodermal cells that later differentiates into the varied endocrine cells of the adenohypophysis. The posterior lobe of the gland (the neurohypophysis) is derived from an out-pouching of the neural ectoderm of the diencephalon of the brain as a result of intrinsic regulation within the forebrain and extrinsic prechordal mesenchymal induction. Rathke's pouch normally loses its connexion with the oral ectoderm by atrophy of the hypophyseal duct and chondrification of the cranial floor during the embryonic

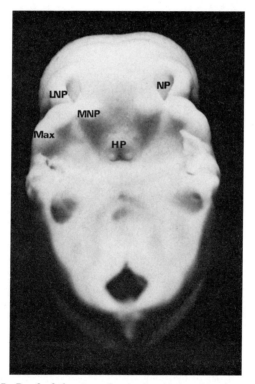

Fig. 37. Roof of the stomodeum of a 41-day-old embryo. The lateral nasal process (LNP) and medial nasal process (MNP) surround the nasal placode (NP) while the hypophyseal pouch (HP) intrudes into the stomodeal roof. The maxillary process (Max) forms the superolateral boundary of the stomodeum. ($\times$17.) (*By courtesy of Professor H. Nishimura.*)

43

period, but if remnants of the duct persist, the basis for *cranio-pharyngeal cysts* or *tumours* within the body of the sphenoid bone exists.

The three sets of facial processes derive their sensory innervation from the three divisions of the trigeminal nerve that develop in the 5th and 6th weeks as part of the full complement of twelve paired cranial nerves. The frontonasal process is innervated by the oph-thalmic division, the maxillary process by the maxillary division, and the mandibular process by the mandibular division of the trigeminal nerve, accounting for the adult pattern of facial sensory nerve supply (*Fig. 39*).

The oral cavity and the entire intestinal tract are sterile at birth. As soon as feeding by mouth commences, an oral bacterial flora

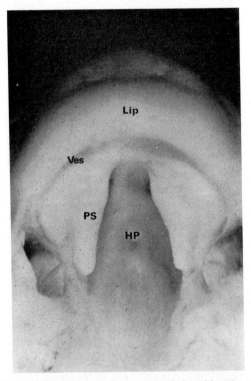

Fig. 38. Roof of the stomodeum of a 54-day-old embryo. The posterior portions of the palatal shelves (**PS**) are in the vertical position while the anterior portions are horizontal. The lip is demarcated from the palate by the vestibular (**Ves**) depression. The remnant of the hypophyseal pouch (**HP**) is seen as a depression in the roof of the stomodeum. (×15.) (*By courtesy of Professor H. Nishimura.*)

44

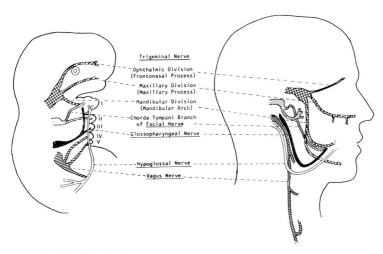

Fig. 39. Distribution of the branches of the trigeminal, facial, glossopharyngeal, hypoglossal and vagal cranial nerves in the fetal and adult head and neck.

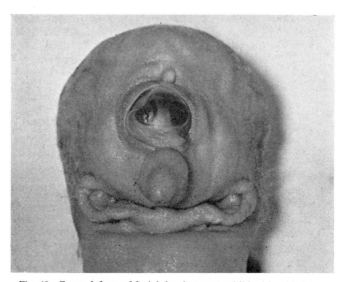

Fig. 40. Gross defects of facial development exhibited by this fetus include fusion of the eyes in the midline to produce cyclopia, protuberant proboscis, synotia, and agnathia. The proboscis is the frontonasal process from which the 'premaxilla' and incisor teeth are regarded as normally developing. The incisors are typically absent in the cyclops.

is established that is to form part of the oral environment throughout life. The oral soft tissues develop a local resistance to infection by the early established bacterial flora that becomes characteristic of the individual mouth.

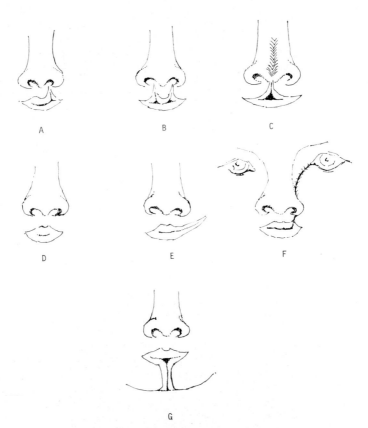

Fig. 41. Defects of orofacial development. A, Unilateral cleft lip. B, Bilateral cleft lip. C, Median cleft lip (true 'hare lip'). D, Microstomia. E, Unilateral macrostomia. F, Unilateral facial cleft. G, Median mandibular cleft.

Defects of Orofacial Development

Gross defects of cranial development, such as *acrania* or *cranioschisis* (a roofless skull), occur with *anencephaly* (absence of brain) and *anophthalmia* (absence of eyes). Lack of development of important organs is generally incompatible with life. Severe local defects, such as location of the eyes to form a single median eye, known as *cyclopia*, and erratic or exuberant growth in the nose region producing proboscis-like masses are often associated with congenital defects in other parts of the body (*Fig. 40*). Other nasal defects include absence of the nose, *arhinia* (no nasal placodes form), and a bifid nose, reflecting a failure of fusion of the medial nasal processes.

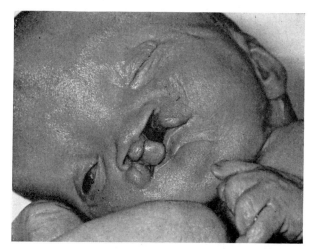

Fig. 42. Newborn infant exhibiting bilateral cleft lip and palate, with consequent projection of the median globular process.

Mild developmental defects of the face are of comparatively common occurrence. Failure of the facial growth centres to merge, or, as it is sometimes termed, failure of fusion of the facial processes, results in abnormal developmental clefts. These clefts are due to disruption of the many integrated processes of induction, cell migration, and mesenchymal merging (*see* p. 109). Unilateral clefting of the upper lip is the result of the globular process failing to merge with the maxillary processes on either side of the midline (*Fig. 41*A). *Unilateral cleft lip*, more usual on the left side, is a relatively common congenital defect (1 in 800 births) that has a strong familial tendency, suggesting a genetic background. The rare *bilateral cleft lip* results in a wide midline defect of the upper lip, and may produce a protuberant proboscis (*Figs. 41*B, *42*). The exceedingly rare *median cleft lip* (a true 'hare-lip') is due to the incomplete merging of the two medial nasal processes into a single globular process. As a consequence, there is also usually an accompanying deep midline grooving of the nose leading to various forms of bifid nose (*Fig. 41*C).

47

Merging of the maxillary and mandibular processes beyond or short of the site for normal mouth size results in either too small a mouth, termed *microstomia** (*Fig. 41*D), or, conversely, too wide a mouth, termed *macrostomia*† (*Fig. 41*E). Rarely, the maxillary and mandibular processes merge completely to produce a closed mouth, termed *astomia*.

An *oblique facial cleft* results from the persistence of the groove between the maxillary process and the lateral nasal process running from the medial canthus of the eye to the ala of the nose (*Fig. 41*F). Persistence of the furrow between the two mandibular processes produces the rare midline *mandibular cleft* (*Fig. 41*G).

Retardation of mandibular development gives rise to *micrognathia* of varying degrees with accompanying dental malocclusion. Total failure of development of the mandible, *agnathia*, is associated with abnormal ventral placement of the external ears (*synotia*) (*Fig. 119*).

Craniofacial developmental cysts, while strictly speaking not a defect of orofacial development, nevertheless have a basis for their origin in the complicated embryonic processes of the craniofacial complex. Developmental cysts arise along the lines of facial and palatal clefts, and their lining epithelia appear to be derived from residues or 'rests' of the covering epithelia of the embryonic processes that merge to form the face. Where such epithelial residues become trapped in the subjacent mesenchyme during merging, or there is an ectopic sequestration of skin or mucosa beneath the surface, a potential for subsequent cyst formation exists. In most instances the subsurface epithelium degenerates, probably by programmed cell death. When such epithelial rests persist, they may be stimulated to proliferate and necrose to produce fluid-filled cysts in postnatal life, after a varying period of dormancy. The nature and cause of developmental-cyst-producing stimuli are unknown. Such cysts tend to be named according to the site in which they develop. Hence, *nasolabial cysts* develop where the lateral nasal process and maxillary process meet; *globulomaxillary cysts* develop more deeply along the line of merging of the globular and maxillary processes. *Median mandibular cysts* develop in the midline site of merging of the two mandibular arches. Cysts of the branchial arches and palate are dealt with respectively in Chapters 5 and 10.

For further discussion of orofacial maldevelopment *see* pp. 85, 109 and 119.

---

*Such microstomial defects are often a feature of syndromes of congenital anomalies of development, among which are trisomy 17–18, craniocarpotarsal syndrome (whistling face), the otopalato-digital syndrome, and occasionally of Turner's syndrome.

†Macrostomia occurs in idiopathic hypercalcaemia, mandibulofacial dysostosis (Treacher-Collins syndrome), and occasionally in Klinefelter's XXY syndrome.

SELECTED BIBLIOGRAPHY

ACKERMAN, J. L. (1965), 'Craniofacial Growth and Development in Cebocephalia', *Oral Surg.*, **19**, 543.

BERGSMA, D. (Ed.) (1975), *Morphogenesis and Malformation of Face and Brain.* New York: Alan R. Liss Inc.

BLECHSCHMIDT, E. (1965), 'Das Antlitz des Menschlichen Embryo', *Die Waage*, **4**, 139.

— — (1968), 'Die Physiognomie in der Embryonalzeit des Menschen', *Ibid.*, **7**, 2.

D'ASSUMPÇAÕ, E. A. (1975), 'Proboscis Lateralis', *Plastic reconstr. Surg.*, **55**, 494.

BIXLER, D., CHRISTIAN, J. C., and GORLIN, R. J. (1969), 'Hypertelorism, Microtia and Facial Clefting: A New Inherited Syndrome', *Birth Defects*, Orig. Art. Series, **5** (2), 77.

BURSTON, W. R., HAMILTON, W. J., and WALKER, D. G. (1964), 'Symposium: Malformation of the Face', *Br. dent. J.*, **116**, 285.

CHANDRA, R., YADAVA, V. N. S., and SHARMA, R. N. (1974), 'Persistent Buccopharyngeal Membrane', *Plastic reconstr. Surg.*, **54**, 678.

DOLLANDER, A. (1977), 'L'Embryologie de la Face', *Actualités Odonto-Stomatologiques*, **120**, 671.

FORRESTER, D. J., CARSTENS, N. K., and SHURTLEFF, D. B. (1966), 'Craniofacial Configuration of Hydrocephalic Children', *J. Am. dent. Ass*, **72**, 1399.

GLASS, D. F. (1970), 'The Recognition of Bilateral Craniofacial Deformities', *Dent. Practnr dent. Rec.*, **21**, 137.

GORDON, H., DAVIES, D., and FRIEDBERG, S. (1969), 'Congenital Pits of the Lower Lip with Cleft Lip and Palate', *S. Afr. med. J.*, **43**, 1275.

HERRING, S. W., ROWLATT, U. F., and PRUZANSKY, S. (1979), 'Anatomical Abnormalities in Mandibulofacial Dysostosis', *Am. J. Med. Gen.*, **3**, 225.

IVY, R. H. (1963), 'Congenital Anomalies', *Plastic reconstr. Surg.*, **32**, 361.

JOHNSTON, M. C., and HAZELTON, R. D., (1972), 'Embryonic Origins of Facial Structures Related to Oral Sensory and Motor Functions', Chapt. 4 in *Third Symposium on Oral Sensation and Perception* (Ed. BOSMA, J. F.). Springfield, Ill.: Thomas.

KNOWLES, C. C., LITTLEWOOD, A. H. M., and BUSH, P. G. (1969), 'Incomplete Median Cleft of the Lower Lip and Chin with Complete Cleft of the Mandible', *Br. dent. J.*, **127**, 337.

KRAUS, B. S., KITAMURA, H., and LATHAM, R. A. (1966), *Atlas of Developmental Anatomy of the Face.* New York: Harper & Row.

KREUTZER, E. W., and JAFEK, B. W. (1980), 'The Vomeronasal Organ of Jacobson in the Human Embryo and Fetus', *Otolaryngol. Head Neck Surg.*, **88**, 119.

LATHAM, R. A. (1971), 'Mechanism of Maxillary Growth in the Human Cyclops', *J. dent. Res.*, **50**, 929.

— — and BURSTON, W. R. (1964), 'The Effect of Unilateral Cleft of the Lip and Palate on Maxillary Growth Pattern', *Br. J. plastic Surg.*, **17**, 10.

MELNICK, M., and JORGENSON, R. (Ed.) (1979), *Developmental Aspects of Craniofacial Dysmorphology*. New York: Alan R. Liss Inc.

MELNICK, M., SHIELDS, E. D., and BURZYNSKI, N. J. (1980), *Clinical Dysmorphology of Oral-Facial Structures*. Littleton, Mass.: Publishing Sciences Group Publication Co.

MOFFETT, B. C. (Ed.), (1972), *Mechanisms and Regulation of Craniofacial Morphogenesis*. Amsterdam: Swets & Zeitlinger.

MONIE, I. W. (1962), 'The Development of the Philtrum', *Plastic reconstr. Surg.*, **30**, 313.

OBWEGESER, H. L., WEBER, G., FREIHOFER, H. P., and SAILER, H., (1978), 'Facial Duplication—the Unique Case of Antonio', *J. Max. Fac. Surg.*, **6**, 179.

PĚNKAVA, J. (1974), 'Median Cleft of the Upper Lip and Jaw', *Acta Chir. Plast.* (*Praha*), **16**, 201.

POWELL, W. J., and JENKINS, H. P. (1968), 'Transverse Facial Clefts', *Plastic reconstr. Surg.*, **42**, 454.

PSAUME, J., and GORLIN, R. J. (1962), 'Orodigitofacial Dysostosis— A New Syndrome', *J. Pediat.*, **61**, 520.

SAKURAI, E. H. (1966), 'Bilateral Oblique Facial Clefts and Amniotic Bands: A Report of Two Cases', *Cleft Palate J.*, **3**, 181.

SCOTT, J. H. (1966), 'The Embryology of Cleft Palate and Hare Lip', *Br. dent. J.*, **120**, 17.

STARK, R. B. (1973), 'Development of the Face', *Surg. Gynecol. Obstet.*, **137**, 403.

VAN OOSTROM, C. G., and VERWOERD, C. D. A. (1972), 'The Origin of the Olfactory Placode', *Acta morph. neerl-scand.*, **9**, 160.

VERMIJ-KEERS, C. (1972), 'Transformations in the Facial Region of the Human Embryo', *Adv. in Anat., Embro. and Cell. Biol.*, **46** (5), 1–30.

VERWOERD, C. D. A., and VAN OOSTROM, C. G. (1979), 'Cephalic Neural Crest and Placodes', *Adv. in Anat., Embryo. and Cell. Biol.*, **58**, 1–75.

VIERS, W. (1973), 'Transmedian Innervation of the Upper Lip: An Embryological Study', *Laryngoscope*, **83**, 1.

WOOD, N. K., WRAGG, L. E., STUTEVILLE, O. H., and KAMINSKI, E. J. (1970), 'Prenatal Observations on the Incisive Fissure and the Frontal Process in Man', *J. dent. Res.*, **49**, 1125.

CHAPTER 4

THE BRANCHIAL ARCHES

DURING the late somite period (4th week i.u.), the mesoderm of the ventral foregut region becomes segmented to form a series of five distinct bilateral mesenchymal swellings, the *branchial (pharyngeal) arches*. The initial mesodermal core of each arch is augmented by later neural crest tissue (ectomesenchyme) invasion that surrounds the mesodermal core. The mesoderm will give rise to muscle myoblasts and endothelial cells, while the neural crest cells give rise to skeletal and connective tissue.

The *branchial arches* are separated by four *branchial grooves* on the external aspect of the embryo, which correspond internally with five outpocketings of the elongated pharynx of the foregut, known as the five *pharyngeal pouches* (*Figs. 43, 44, 45*). The appearance of these temporary structures in the embryo has been likened to the gill arches and clefts of fishes, as an example of vertebrate evolution being recapitulated in embryonic development.* However, unlike the gill clefts of fishes, the grooves of the human embryo are never open, and the ecto-meso-endodermal membranes between the branchial arches remain intact (*Fig. 45*). Neural crest cells migrate into the branchial arches beneath their epithelial covering and surround the mesoderm of each arch.

The branchial arch sizes decrease in craniocaudal sequence from the first to the sixth† each pair merging midventrally to form semicircular 'collars' around the pharynx. Only five pairs of arches are discernible, however, the fifth being transitory. Each pair of arches develops a basic, phylogenetically old set of structures that are adapted to new uses in later ontogenetic development. In each of the five pairs of arches are (*Figs. 45, 46*):

1. A central *cartilage rod* that forms the skeleton of the arch.
2. A muscular component, termed a *branchiomere*.
3. A vascular component, consisting of an *aortic arch artery* running around the pharynx from the ventrally located heart to the dorsal aorta.

---

*This phenomenon was postulated as part of an 'ontogeny recapitulates phylogeny' hypothesis, now discredited, proposed by Haeckel (1866), wherein he theorized that a developing individual (ontogeny) goes through the same changes, in a condensed form, as the species did when evolving (phylogeny). Phylogenetically old structures may be converted to new uses, or phylogenetically newer structures may utilize components of older ones during early embryonic (ontogenetic) development.

†The last arch is labelled the sixth since structures derived from it are homologous with sixth arch derivatives of lower vertebrates.

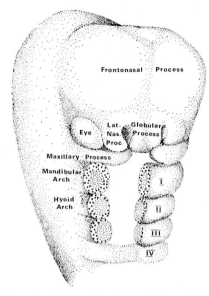

Fig. 43. Schematic diagram of embryo with a section of the first three branchial arches cut away, revealing the invading neural crest mesenchyme (large dots) surrounding the mesodermal core. (*By courtesy of Dr M. C. Johnston*, 1972, *in* Cleft Lip and Palate. *Baltimore: Williams & Wilkins.*)

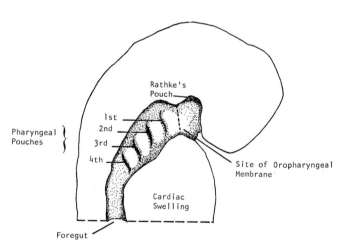

Fig. 44. Internal representation of the pharyngeal pouches (numbered) in a somite period embryo.

4. A nervous element, consisting of sensory and special visceral motor fibres of one or more cranial nerves supplying the mucosa and branchial muscle arising from that arch.

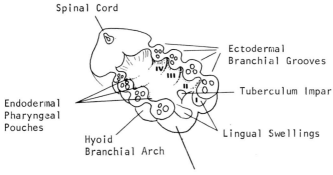

Spinal Cord

Ectodermal Branchial Grooves

Endodermal Pharyngeal Pouches

Tuberculum Impar

Hyoid Branchial Arch

Lingual Swellings

Mandibular Branchial Arch

Fig. 45. Schema of early branchial arch development. Branchial arches numbered in Roman numerals. (*After Waterman and Meller.*)

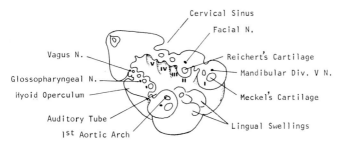

Cervical Sinus

Facial N.

Vagus N.

Reichert's Cartilage

Glossopharyngeal N.

Mandibular Div. V N.

Hyoid Operculum

Meckel's Cartilage

Auditory Tube

1st Aortic Arch

Lingual Swellings

Fig. 46. Schema of later branchial arch development. Branchial arches numbered in Roman numerals. (*After Waterman and Meller.*)

The cartilage rods, which are differentiated from neural crest tissue that has been organized by pharyngeal endoderm, are variously adapted to bony, cartilaginous or ligamentous structures, or in some cases may disappear in later development. The branchiomeric muscle components are of lateral plate mesoderm origin, giving rise to special visceral muscles that, though not of somitic origin, are composed of striated muscle fibres.* Nerve fibres of specific cranial

*The striated (voluntary) branchial arch musculature is a phylogenetic secondary adaptation of the initially smooth (involuntary) visceral muscles of the branchial arches. A remnant of this historical derivation is retained in the smooth muscle of the orbit that is presumed to be of first branchial arch origin. This smooth muscle (of Müller) that is embryologically part of the masticatory musculature spans the inferior orbital fissure.

Table I.—Derivatives of the Branchial Arches, Pharyngeal Pouches and Cranial Somites

Branchial Arch	Endodermal Pouch	Branchial Arch Arteries	Branchiomeric Muscle	Efferent Nerve	Skeleton (Viscerocranium)
1st Mandibular	★(D)Tubotympanic recess, which forms *auditory tube* and *middle ear cavity* †(V)Obliterated by tongue	Contributes to *external carotid* and *maxillary arteries*	*Muscles of mastication* (temporal, masseter, and pterygoids) mylohyoid, ant. digastric, *tensor veli palatini, tensor tympani*	V *Mandibular nerve* motor branch	Maxillary process and palatal shelf, Incus, spine of sphenoid bone Malleus, anterior ligament of malleus, sphenomand. lig. and core of mandible from Meckel's cartilage
2nd Hyoid	★(D)Mostly filled in by own proliferation to form *tonsillar fossa* and *palatine tonsil* ★(V)Obliterated by tongue	*Stapedial artery* (in part) possibly small contribution to *facial artery*	*Muscles of facial expression,* posterior digastric, stylohyoid, stapedius	VII *Facial nerve*	Stapes, styloid process, stylohyoid ligament, lesser horn and upper part of *hyoid body* (Reichert's cartilage)
3rd	★(D)Parathyroid III (inferior) †(V)Thymus	*Proximal 1/3 of internal carotid,* possibly small contribution to *common carotid*	*Stylopharyngeus* ? upper pharyngeal muscles	IX *Glossopharyngeal nerve* (pharyngeal plexus)	*Greater horn* and lower part of *hyoid body*
4th	★(D)Parathyroid IV †(V)Lateral thyroid Vestigial thymus	*Arch of aorta* (left) Proximal part of *right subclavian* (right)	*Pharyngeal constrictors* ? Levator palatini, Cricothyroid and Laryngeal muscles ? Palatoglossus	X *Superior laryngeal nerve* (pharyngeal plexus)	*Thyroid and laryngeal cartilages*

Table I (continued)

Branchial Arch	Endodermal Pouch	Branchial Arch Arteries	Branchiomeric Muscle	Efferent Nerve	Skeleton (Viscerocranium)
5th	Ultimobranchial body or cyst (sometimes)	Nothing—rarely seen	Same as 4th branchial arch		*Lower part thyroid cartilage and laryngeal cartilages*
6th	None	Proximal part of both *pulmonary arteries* and most of *ductus arteriosus* (left)	Laryngeal muscles except cricothyroid	X *Inferior laryngeal nerve*	*Cricoid cartilage* (probably)
Postbranchial region			Trapezius Sternomastoid	XI Spinal accessory	Tracheal cartilages??
SOMITES			MYOTOMIC MUSCLE		SCLEROTOMES
4 Occipital Somites			Intrinsic tongue muscles Styloglossus } Extrinsic Hyoglossus tongue Genioglossus muscles	XII Hypoglossal	Basi-occipital bone
Prechordal Somites			?Extrinsic ocular muscles	III, Oculomotor IV, Trochlear VI, Abducens	Nasal capsule? Nasal septum?
Upper Cervical Somites			Geniohyoid; Infrahyoid muscles	Spinal nerves C1, 2	Cervical vertebrae

55

*(D) = Dorsal.
†(V) = Ventral.

nerves enter the mesoderm of the branchial arches, initiating muscle development in the branchiomeric mesoderm. The muscles arising from the mesodermal 'cores' adapt to the branchial arch derivatives, and migrate from their sites of origin. The original nerve-supply to these muscles is maintained during migration, accounting for the devious routes of many cranial nerves in adult anatomy. The blood vascular system originates from lateral plate mesoderm. The arteries are modified from their symmetrical primitive embryonic pattern, reminiscent of that in aquatic vertebrates, into the asymmetrical form of the adult derivatives of the fourth and sixth arch arteries.

First Branchial Arch

The first or mandibular pair of branchial arches are the precursors of the jaws, both maxillary and mandibular, and appropriately bound the lateral aspects of the stomodeum, at this stage merely a depression in the early facial region. The maxilla is derived from a small *maxillary process* extending cranioventrally from the much larger mandibular branchial arch. The cartilage skeleton of the first arch is known as *Meckel's cartilage* (*Fig. 46*) arising at the 41st to 45th days i.u. provides a template for subsequent development of the mandible, but most of its cartilage substance disappears in the formed mandible. The mental ossicle is the only portion of the mandible derived from Meckel's cartilage by endochondral ossification.

Persisting portions of Meckel's cartilage form the basis of major portions of two ear ossicles, the *malleus** and *incus,*† the *spine of the sphenoid bone*, and two ligaments—the *anterior ligament of the malleus* and the *sphenomandibular ligament*. The branchiomeric musculature of the mandibular arch subdivides and migrates to form the *muscles of mastication*, the *mylohyoid muscle*, the *anterior belly of the digastric*, the *tensor tympani*‡ and the *tensor veli palatini muscles*, all of which are innervated by the nerve of the first arch, viz., the *mandibular division of the Vth cranial* or *trigeminal nerve* (*Fig. 46*). The sensory component of this nerve innervates the mandible and its covering mucosa and gingiva, the mandibular teeth, the mucosa of the anterior two-thirds of the tongue, the floor of the mouth, and the skin of the lower third of the face. The first arch artery contributes, in part, to the *maxillary artery* and to a portion of the *external carotid artery*.

---

*The anterior process of the malleus forms independently in membrane bone.
†The incus arises from the separated end of Meckel's cartilage that corresponds with the pterygo-quadrate cartilage of inframammalian vertebrates.
‡The tensor tympani is the evolutionary remnant of a reptilian jaw muscle attached to the remnant of the reptilian jaw, i.e. Meckel's cartilage.

Second Branchial Arch

The cartilage of the second or *hyoid arch* (Reichert's cartilage) appearing at the 45th to 48th days i.u. is the basis of the greater part (head, neck, and crura) of the third ear ossicle, the *stapes*,* and contributes to the malleus and incus,† the *styloid process* of the temporal bone, the *stylohyoid ligament*, and the *lesser horn* and cranial part of the *body of the hyoid bone* (*Fig. 47*).

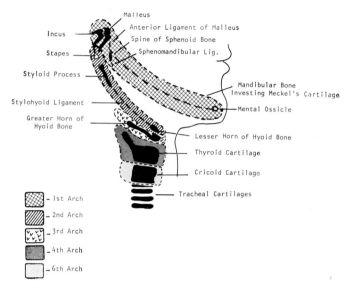

Fig. 47. Schema of the adult derivatives of the branchial arches. Note that the malleus, incus, and hyoid bones are each derived from two branchial arches.

The branchiomeric muscles of the hyoid arch subdivide and migrate extensively to form the *stapedius*, the *stylohyoid*, the *posterior belly of the digastric* and all the *mimetic muscles* of the face, all of which are innervated by the *VIIth cranial* or *facial nerve*, serving the second arch. The paths of migration of these muscles are traced out in the adult by the distribution of branches of the facial nerve. The special sensory component of this nerve for taste, known as the *chorda tympani* nerve, invades the first branchial arch as a pretrematic nerve and thus comes to supply the mucosa of the anterior

---

*The footplate of the stapes is derived in part from the otic capsule.

†The manubrium of the malleus and the long crus of the incus are of second arch derivation.

two-thirds of the tongue. The artery of this arch forms the *stapedial artery** that disappears during the fetal period, leaving the foramen in the stapes.

Third Branchial Arch

The cartilage of this small arch produces the *greater horn* and caudal part of the *body of the hyoid bone*. The remainder of the cartilage disappears. The branchial musculature forms the *stylopharyngeus muscle*, innervated by the *IXth (glossopharyngeal) nerve* supplying the arch. The mucosa of the posterior one-third of the tongue is derived from this arch, which accounts for its sensory innervation by the glossopharyngeal nerve.

The artery of this arch contributes to the *common carotid* and part of the *internal carotid arteries*.

Fourth Branchial Arch

The cartilage of this arch probably forms the thyroid cartilage. The branchiomeric muscles develop into the *cricothyroid* and *constrictors of the pharynx*, the *levator veli palatini* and *uvular* muscles of the soft palate, and the *palatoglossus muscle* of the tongue. The nerve of the fourth arch is the *superior laryngeal branch of the vagus*, or *Xth cranial nerve* that innervates these muscles.

The fourth arch artery of the left side forms the arch of the *aorta*; that of the right side contributes to the *right subclavian* and *brachiocephalic* arteries.

Fifth Branchial Arch

The fifth branchial arch is a transitory structure that disappears almost as soon as it forms, and bequeaths no permanent structural elements.

Sixth Branchial Arch

The cartilage of this arch probably forms the *cricoid* and *arytenoid* cartilages of the larynx. The branchiomeric muscle forms the *intrinsic muscles of the larynx*, which are supplied by the nerve of the arch, the *recurrent laryngeal branch of the Xth cranial* or *vagus nerve*. Because the nerve of this arch passes caudal to the fourth arch artery in its recurring path from the brain to the muscles it supplies, the differing fate of the left and right fourth arch arteries, when migrating caudally into the thorax, accounts for the different recurrent paths of the left and right laryngeal nerves. The right recurrent laryngeal nerve recurves around the right subclavian artery, while the left laryngeal nerve recurves around the aorta.

---

*The stapedial artery, a branch of the internal carotid artery, initially supplies the deep portion of the face, an area that is taken over by branches of the external carotid artery once the stapedial artery disappears.

The sixth arch arteries develop in part into the *pulmonary arteries*, the remainder disappearing on the right side, and on the left side, forming the temporary *ductus arteriosus* of the fetal circulation.

Postbranchial Region

Controversy surrounds the embryological origin of the tracheal cartilages and the sternomastoid and trapezius muscles. On the basis of their nerve supply (spinal accessory cranial nerve XI), it appears that the latter two muscles are of mixed somitic and branchial origin.

The Hyoid Bone

This composite* endochondral bone derived from the cartilages of the second (hyoid) and third branchial arches reflects its double origin in its six centres of ossification, two for the body, one for each lesser horn, and one for each greater horn. Ossification centres for the greater horns appear at the end of fetal life (38 weeks), those for the body at about birth and those for the lesser horns at about 2 years postnatally. The lesser horns may not fuse with the body, but attach by fibrous tissue to the major horns that in turn articulate with the body through a diarthrodial synovial joint. The double origin of the hyoid body, from the second and third branchial arches, is very occasionally reflected as a bone split into upper and lower portions. Fusion of all these elements into a single bone occurs late in post-natal life.

SELECTED BIBLIOGRAPHY

BARRY, A. (1961), 'Development of the Branchial Region of Human Embryos with Special Reference to the Fate of the Epithelia', in *Congenital Anomalies of the Face and Associated Structures* (Ed. PRUZANSKY, S.). Springfield, Ill.: Thomas.

HAST, M. H. (1972), 'Early Development of the Human Laryngeal Muscles', *Trans. Am. Laryngol. Assoc.*, 93rd Mtg, pp. 27–34.

HERRMANN, J., and OPITZ, J. M. (1969), 'A Dominantly Inherited First Arch Syndrome', *Birth Defects*, Orig. Art. Series, 5 (2), 110.

KARMODY, C. S., and FEINGOLD, M. (1974), 'Autosomal Dominant First and Second Branchial Arch Syndrome', in *Malformation Syndromes* (Ed. BERGSMA, D.) 10, 31. New York: International Medical Book Corp.

---

*The hyoid bone consists of several independent elements that, although fused together in man, remain separate in many animals as the 'hyoid apparatus'. Of these separate elements, the typanohyal and stylohyal form the styloid process in man. The ceratohyal forms the lesser horn and upper part of the body of the human hyoid. The epihyal does not form a bone in man, but is incorporated into the stylohyoid ligament. The thyrohyal that develops from the 3rd arch forms the greater horn and lower part of the body of the human hyoid bone.

KOEBKE, J. (1978), 'Some Observations on the Development of the Human Hyoid Bone', *Anat. Embryol.*, **153**, 279.

McKENZIE, J. (1966), 'The First Arch Syndrome', *Devl med. Child. Neurol.*, **8**, 55.

POSWILLO, D. (1973), 'The Pathogenesis of the First and Second Branchial Arch Syndrome', *Oral Surg.*, **35**, 302.

RICHANY, S. F., BAST, T. H., and ANSON, B. J. (1956), 'The Development of the First Branchial Arch in Man and the Fate of Meckel's Cartilage', *Q. Bull. NWest. Univ. med. Sch.*, **30**, 331.

TRAIL, M. L., LYONS, G. D., and CREELY, J. J. (1972), 'Anomalies of the First Branchial Cleft', *South. Med. J.*, **65**, 716.

CHAPTER 5

THE PHARYNGEAL POUCHES AND
BRANCHIAL GROOVES

THE primitive pharynx forms in the late embryonic period as a
dilatation of the cranial end of the foregut, lying between the developing heart anteriorly and the developing chondrocranium postero-
superiorly. The early pharynx is large relative to the rest of the
gut, is flattened anteroposteriorly and gives rise to a number of
diverse structures derived from its floor and side walls. The lateral
aspects of the comparatively elongated primitive pharynx project
a series of pouches between the branchial arches, the *pharyngeal
pouches*, that sequentially decrease in size craniocaudally (*Fig. 48*).
Intervening between the branchial arches externally are the *branchial grooves* (ectodermal clefts) (*see Figs. 43, 44,* p. 52). The lining
of the branchial grooves is the surface ectoderm, while foregut
endoderm lines the internal pharyngeal pouches (*see Fig. 45,* p. 53).
Each ectodermal branchial groove corresponds with each endodermal pharyngeal pouch with a layer of mesenchyme intervening
between the outer and inner primary germ layers.

The endodermal lining of the primitive pharynx gradually develops
from a polyhedral cuboidal embryonic epithelium into a respiratory

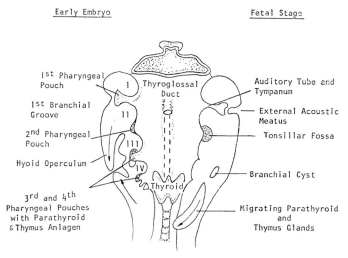

Fig. 48. Schema of pharyngeal pouch and branchial groove
development.

61

mucous membrane, characterized by a ciliated columnar epithelium and goblet cells.

The first branchial groove persists and deepens to form the *external acoustic meatus*. The ecto-meso-endodermal membrane in the depth of the groove, separating it from the first pharyngeal pouch, persists as the *tympanic membrane* (*Fig. 49*). Subsequent external and middle ear development is described in Chapter 18 (*q.v.*).

The second, third, and fourth branchial grooves become obliterated by the caudal overgrowth of the second branchial arch (*hyoid operculum*), which provides a smooth contour to the neck. Failure to obliterate completely these branchial grooves results in a *branchial fistula* leading from the pharynx to the outside, or a *branchial (cervical) sinus or cyst*, forming a closed sac (*Fig. 48*).

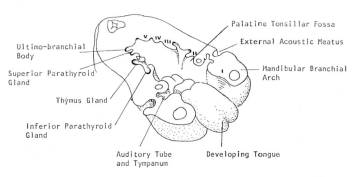

Fig. 49. Schema of derivatives of the pharyngeal pouches. (*After Waterman and Meller.*)

The five pairs of pharyngeal pouches on the sides of the pharyngeal foregut form dorsal and ventral pockets, of which the endodermal epithelium differentiates into a variety of structures. Elongation of the third, fourth and fifth pharyngeal pouches during the 6th and 7th weeks i.u. increasingly dissociates the pouches from the pharynx, and allows their derivatives to form in the lower anterior neck region.

First Pharyngeal Pouch

The ventral portion of this pouch is obliterated by the developing tongue. The dorsal diverticulum deepens laterally as the *tubotympanic recess* to form the *auditory tube*, widening at its end into the *tympanum* or middle ear cavity, separated from the first branchial groove by the *tympanic membrane*. The tympanum becomes occupied by the dorsal ends of the cartilages of the first and second branchial arches that later develop into the ear ossicles. The tympanum maintains contact with the pharynx via the auditory tube throughout life.

The proximal portion of the auditory tube becomes lined with respiratory mucous membrane, and fibrous tissue and cartilage form in its walls. The changing location of the site of opening of the auditory tube reflects the growth of the nasopharynx. The opening is inferior to the hard palate in the fetus, is level with it at birth, and well above the hard palate in the adult.

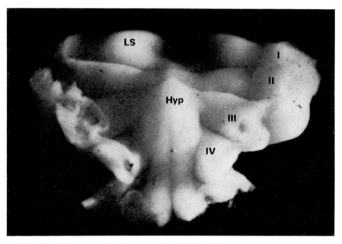

Fig. 50. The ventral pharyngeal wall of a 32-day-old embryo. The branchial arches are marked I–IV. The lingual swellings (LS) are rising from the first branchial arches. The hypobranchial eminence (Hyp) forms a prominent central elevation from which the epiglottis will arise. ($\times$ 41.) (*By courtesy of Professor H. Nishimura.*)

Second Pharyngeal Pouch

The ventral portion of this pouch is obliterated by the developing tongue. The dorsal portion of this pouch persists in an attenuated form as the *tonsillar fossa*, the endodermal lining of which covers the underlying mesodermal lymphatic tissue to form the *palatine tonsil*.*

Third Pharyngeal Pouch

The ventral diverticulum endoderm proliferates and migrates from

---

*It should be noted that neither the pharyngeal nor lingual tonsils are of pharyngeal pouch origin.

each side to form the single median *thymus* gland. The dorsal diverticulum endoderm differentiates and migrates caudally to form the *inferior parathyroid gland*. The glands derived from the endodermal lining of the pouch lose their connexion with the pharyngeal wall when the pouches become obliterated during later development.

Fourth Pharyngeal Pouch

The fate of the endoderm of the ventral diverticulum is uncertain. The lining membrane may possibly contribute to thymus or thyroid tissue.

The dorsal diverticulum endoderm differentiates into the *superior parathyroid gland*, which after losing contact with the pharynx, migrates caudally with the thyroid gland.

Fifth Pharyngeal Pouch

The attenuated fifth pharyngeal pouch appears as a diverticulum of the fourth pouch, the endoderm of which forms the *ultimobranchial body*. The calcitonin-secreting cells of the ultimobranchial body, however, are derived from neural crest tissue and are eventually incorporated into the thyroid gland.

SELECTED BIBLIOGRAPHY

ARNOT, R. S. (1971), 'Defects of the First Branchial Cleft', *S. Afr. J. Surg.*, **9**, 93.

BOYSEN, M. E., DE BESCHE, A., DJUPESLAND, G., and THORUD, E., (1979), 'Internal Cysts and Fistulae of Branchial Origin', *J. Laryngol. and Otol.*, **93**, 533.

CALONIUS, P. E. B., HAKALA, P., and RAPOLA, J. (1974), 'Congenital Cervical Cysts and Fistulas', *Proc. Finn. Dent. Soc.*, **70**, 209.

CASTELLI, W. A., RAMIREZ, P. C., and NASJLETI, C. E. (1973), 'Linear Growth Study of the Pharyngeal Cavity', *J. dent. Res.*, **52**, 1245.

FRASER, B. A., and DUCKWORTH, J. W. A. (1979), 'Ultimobranchial Body Cysts in the Human Foetal Thyroid: Pathological Implications', *J. Pathol.*, **127**, 89.

FRAZER, J. E. (1910), 'The Early Development of the Eustachian Tube and Nasopharynx', *Br. med. J.*, **2**, 1148.

GRIFFIN, C. J., and MCGRATH, P. (1978), *Embryogenesis, Development and Some Anomalies of the Upper Respiratory Tract Including the Septomaxillary Syndrome and its Treatment.* Sydney: Sydney University Press.

KARMODY, C. S. (1979), 'A Classification of the Anomalies of the First Branchial Groove', *Otolaryngol. Head Neck Surg.*, **87**, 334.

KANAGASUNTHERAM, R., and RAMSBOTHAM, M. (1968), 'Development of the Human Nasopharyngeal Epithelium', *Acta anat.*, **70**, 1.

MAUE-DICKSON, W., DICKSON, D. R., and ROOD, S. R. (1976), 'Anatomy of the Eustachian Tube and Related Structures in Age-matched Human Fetuses with and without Cleft Palate', *Trans. Am. Acad. Ophthalmol. Otolaryngol.*, **82**, 159.

PEARSE, A. G. E., and POLAK, J. M. (1971), 'Cytochemical Evidence for the Neural Crest Origin of Mammalian Ultimobranchial C Cells', *Histochemie*, **27**, 96.

POULSEN, J., and TOS, M. (1975), 'Goblet Cells in the Developing Human Nose', *Acta Otolaryngol.*, **80**, 434.

SUGIYAMA, S. (1969), 'Embryonic Development of Human Thyroid Gland and Ultimobranchial Body', *Acta Endocrinol. Copenh.*, Suppl., **138**, 179.

TOS, M. (1971), 'Growth of the Foetal Eustachian Tube and its Dimensions', *Arch. Klin. Exp. Ohren Nasen Kehlkopfheilkd.*, **198**, 177.

— —(1975), 'Goblet Cells in the Developing Rhinopharynx and Pharynx', *Arch. Oto-Rhino- Laryng.*, **209**, 315.

TUCKER, J. A., and O'RAHILLY, R. O. (1972), 'Observations on the Embryology of the Human Larynx', *Trans. Am. Laryngol. Assoc.*, 93rd Mtg, pp. 35–38.

— — and TUCKER, G. F. (1975), 'Some Aspects of Fetal Laryngeal Development', *Ann. Otol.*, **84**, 49.

VIDIĆ, B. (1971), 'The Morphogenesis of the Lateral Nasal Wall in the Early Prenatal Life of Man', *Am. J. Anat.*, **130**, 121.

WEITZNER, S. (1970), 'Branchial Cyst of Oropharynx', *Oral Surg.*, **30**, 607.

WIND, J. (1970), *On the Phylogeny and Ontogeny of the Human Larynx*. Groningen: Wolters-Noordhoff Publ.

CHAPTER 6

CHARACTERISTICS OF BONE DEVELOPMENT AND GROWTH

BONE formation occurs by two methods of differentiation of mesenchymal tissue that may be of mesodermal or ectomesenchymal (neural crest) origin. Accordingly, two varieties of ossification are described. The transformation of mesenchymal connective tissue, usually in membranous sheets, into osseous tissue is known as *intramembranous ossification*, while the conversion of hyaline cartilage prototype models into bone is described as *endochondral ossification*. The adult structure of the osseous tissue formed by the two methods is indistinguishable, and the two methods can be utilized in the formation of what may eventually become a single bone, with the distinctions of its different origins effaced. In the main, the long bones of the limbs and the bones of the thoracic cage and cranial base are generally of endochondral origin, while those of the vault of the skull, the mandible, and clavicle are predominantly of intramembranous origin. Membrane bones appear to be of neural crest origin, and arise after the ectomesenchyme interacts with an epithelium.

Endochondral bone is three-dimensional in its grown pattern, ossifying from one or more deeply seated and slowly expanding centres. The interstitial growth expansion capability of cartilage, even under weight pressure, due to its avascularity precluding pressure ischaemia,* allows for directed prototype cartilage growth. The cartilage 'template' is then replaced by endochondral bone, accounting for indirect bone growth. Intramembranous bone growth, by contrast, is by direct deposition of osseous tissue in osteogenic (periosteal) membranes creating accretional growth, often with great speed, especially over rapidly growing areas, such as the frontal lobes of the brain, or at fracture sites.

Certain inherited congenital defects of bone formation are confined to one or the other type of ossification. Thus, the condition of achondroplasia affects only bones of endochondral origin, while the condition of cleidocranial dysostosis afflicts only those bones of intramembranous origin. On the other hand, the inherited condition of osteogenesis imperfecta afflicts the whole skeleton, whether of endochondral or intramembranous origin.

---

*Cartilage nutrition is provided by perfusing tissue fluids that are not easily obstructed by load pressures.

Ossification commences at definable points in either membranes or cartilages, from which *centres of ossification*★ the ossifying process radiates into the precursor membrane or cartilage. Secondary cartilages, not part of the cartilaginous primordium of the embryo, appear in certain membrane bones (mandible, clavicle) after intramembranous ossification begins. Endochondral ossification occurs later in these secondary cartilages of intramembranous bone. The distinction between intramembranous and endochondral bone, while useful at the embryological level of osteogenesis, tends to become insignificant in postnatal life. As an example, during repair of fractures of intramembranous bone, cartilage may appear in the healing callus, thereby contradicting its embryological origins. Further, the subsequent remodelling of initially endochondral bones by surface resorption and deposition by the membranous periosteum or endosteum effectively replaces most endochondral bone with intramembranous bone. Consequently, most endochondral bones become a blended combination of endochondral and intramembranous components.

In the fetus or postnatally, a *primary centre of ossification* is the first to appear, and this may be later followed by one or more *secondary centres*, all of which coalesce into a single bone. Most primary ossification centres appear before birth, while secondary centres appear postnatally. There is evidence of an osteogenesis-inhibiting mechanism located in embryonic sutural tissue, accounting for the development of discrete bones. Separate bones may fuse into a single composite bone, either as a phylogenetic phenomenon, exemplified in the cranial base, or as an ontogenetic phenomenon, exemplified in the several bones of the skull calvaria fusing into a single bone in extreme old age.

Details of the mechanisms of ossification and the processes of calcification, deposition, and resorption of bone through the operation of osteoblasts and osteoclasts are best studied in histology and physiology texts. The dependence of osseous tissue upon calcium and phosphate metabolism results in the structure of bone being a highly sensitive indicator of the state of turnover of these and other bone minerals. Moreover, bone growth, maintenance, repair, and degeneration depend upon the actions of certain hormones and vitamins operating either indirectly through control of calcium and phosphate and general metabolism, or directly by their varying influences on growth cartilages. Appreciation of these complex physiological and biochemical phenomena is necessary for a full understanding of the mechanisms of morphogenesis of adult bone

---

★A completely accurate timetable of the onset of prenatal ossification of all bones is still not available.

structure and shape, but a discussion of this is outside the scope of the present work.*

The basic shape, and to a considerable degree, the size of bones are genetically determined. Once this inherited fundamental morphology is established, environmentally variable minor features of bones, such as ridges etc. develop. Superimposed upon the basic bone architecture are nutritional, hormonal, and functional influences that, because of the slow and continual replacement of osseous tissue occurring throughout life, enable bones to respond morphologically to functional stresses. Specific periosteal and capsular functional matrices (*see* p. 5) influence specific portions of related bones termed *skeletal units*. Macroskeletal units may consist of a single bone, or of adjacent portions of several bones, e.g., the frontal, parietal and temporal bones of the calvaria. Each macroskeletal unit is made up of microskeletal units that respond independently to functional matrices and thereby determine the varying shapes of the macroskeletal unit or classically-named bone. While the specific growth rates of the individual microskeletal units might differ from one another, there is, none the less, a constant proportionality between growth rates, thereby imparting a fairly constant shape to the enlarging macroskeletal unit.

Based upon the influence of muscles on bone morphology, three classes of morphological features of the craniofacial skeleton have been identified: (1) those that never appear unless muscles are present, e.g., temporal line, nuchal lines; (2) those that are self-differentiating but require the presence of muscles to persist, e.g., angular process of mandible, and (3) those that are largely independent of the muscles with which they are associated, e.g., the zygomatic bone or the body of the mandible.

The exact mechanism by which functional deforming mechanical forces produce structural bone changes is obscure, but it appears to be mediated through piezo-electric currents. Bone, being so highly crystalline due to its collagen and apatite content, behaves as a crystal by generating a minute electric current when it is mechanically deformed, thereby producing polar electric fields. Bioelectric effects may be generated in several ways, and electrical potential differences are a feature of all cell membranes. It is conceivable that osteoclasts and osteoblasts and the matrix within which they operate react to electric potentials by building up bone (experiments suggest) in negatively charged fields, and conversely, resorbing bone in positively charged fields. These stress potential currents may

---

*An additional factor of significance in bone physiology and morphology is its haemopoietic function. Bone marrow haemopoiesis begins in the 3rd month i.u., and rapidly replaces liver haemopoiesis as the most important site for blood cell formation.

allow for the adjustments in bone structure that are made to meet new functional demands.

In orthodontics, distinction is made between genetically-determined unalterable 'basal' bone and the superimposed 'functional' bone that is amenable to manipulated alteration. In practice, 'basal' bone refers to the body of the maxilla or mandible, while 'functional' bone is the alveolar bone of both jaws that supports the teeth and which responds to orthodontic forces. The ultimate shape of a bone and its internal architecture, then, is a reflection of its inherited form and the mechanical demands to which it is subjected. Intrinsic genetic factors may only play an initial role in determining the size, shape and growth of a bone. Extrinsic functional or environmental factors become the predominant determinator of bone form. Since the environment is constantly changing, bones never attain a 'final' morphology, and their shapes are continually subject to change. It has been observed that a bone is composed of the minimum quantity of osseous tissue that will successfully withstand the usual functional stresses applied to it. This supposedly accounts for the hollow marrow centres of long bones and possibly the presence of sinuses in the skull bones. These factors were formulated into a trajectorial theory of bone structure by Culmann and Meyer just after the middle of the last century and proposed as Wolff's Law (1870) stating that changes in the function of a bone are attended by alterations in its structure.

During adolescence there is a spurt in bone growth that is believed to be mediated by circulating growth hormones. Bones may differ in the timing of their maximum increases within individuals, suggesting that intrinsic factors in different skull bones may be important in determining changes in the rate of growth at different ages. Circulating growth hormones do not alone determine the timing of the adolescent growth spurt. The pattern of timing of variations in bone growth velocity is intrinsically, and presumably genetically, determined. Hormones augment a genetically regulated pattern of growth rate in the cranial base.

An interposed cartilage (i.e., an epiphysis)* converting to osseous tissue adds to an endochondral bone's length and simultaneously actively displaces adjacent parts of the bone by expansion in opposite directions. Embryonic cartilage cells are haphazardly arranged, precluding directionality of growth. By contrast, specialized (epiphyseal) growth plates contain organized columns of cartilage

---

*The bones of teleost fishes do not have cartilaginous growth plates. Appositional growth of their bones has no limit. Amphibians and reptiles possess cartilaginous epiphyses that persist throughout life, providing for potentially continuous growth. The osseous fusion of mammalian epiphyses limits the growth potential of their bones.

Modes of Growth

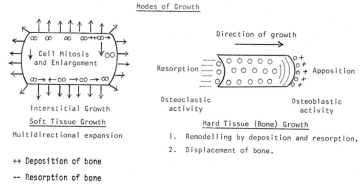

Fig. 51. Modes of growth.

cells, accounting for highly directed growth. The growth forces originate for the most part within the bone's cartilage. On the other hand, most intramembranous bones with sutural contacts become separated by external, capsular functional matrix growth forces (e.g., the expanding brain or eyeball). Addition of osseous tissue to these membranous sutural surfaces passively fills in the widened interval in a field of tension, contrasting with the compression field created by the endochondral mechanism.

The overall growth of bones, resulting in their recognizable expansion, is a function of two phenomena, viz., remodelling and transposition. Remodelling is a combination of accretional growth and resorption of bone and is a response, in part at least, to periosteal functional matrices. Because of the rigid nature of calcified bone, intrinsic growth of this tissue must necessarily be appositional, by cortical surface deposition of newly-formed bone. This primary mode of bone growth is in contrast to the interstitial form of growth that takes place in most soft tissues, which can expand in size by division and growth of cells within the tissue (*Fig. 51*). Such internal expansion is not possible in rigid bone. Concomitant with the deposition of bone in certain areas, resorption occurs in other areas to allow for remodelling, i.e., changing the shape of a bone. The periosteum covering the surface of bone provides a ready source of osteoblasts for deposition and osteoclasts for resorption. The rate of remodelling diminishes when growth slows down, and bone density increases.

The second basic phenomenon of bone growth, viz., transposition, is displacement of the remodelling bones *vis-à-vis* each other. Bone displacement is the result of forces exerted by the surrounding soft tissues (capsular matrices) and by the primary intrinsic growth of the

70

bones themselves. Bone growth as a whole accordingly represents the cumulative effects of intrinsic remodelling (a vector of deposition and resorption) and displacement. These several phenomena may occur in the same or in diverse directions, but their combination is usually a complex one, and their relative contributions are difficult to determine. This difficulty is the source of much controversy relating to craniofacial bone growth.

Bone Articulations

Since the sites of junction between bones, known as articulations or joints, play an important role in bone growth phenomena, it is useful here to classify bony articulations.

A. Movable Joints (Diarthroses)

All movable joints are characterized by the presence of a synovial membrane lining a joint cavity. Different varieties of synovial joints are classified according to the shapes of the participating bones, e.g., ball and socket joints, or the nature of their action, e.g., hinge joints.

B. Immovable Joints (Synarthroses)

Junctional tissue	Articulation type	Example
Fibrous connective tissue	Syndesmosis	Skull suture
Cartilage	Synchondrosis	Symphysis pubis
Bone	Synostosis	Symphysis menti

Diarthroses, per se, do not play a significant role in bone growth except in the temporomandibular joint. The articular cartilage of the temporomandibular joint alone, of all the articular cartilages, provides a growth potential for one of the articulating bones, viz., the mandible. All other articular cartilages are inactive in the growth phenomena of their associated bones.

Synarthroses, on the other hand, play a very significant part in the growth of the articulating bones.

The apposition of bone during growth may take two forms:

(a) *Surface deposition*, accounting for increased thickness of bone that may be modified in remodelling by selective resorption.

(b) *Sutural deposition*, restricted to the opposing edges of bones at a suture site, and accounting for the 'filling in' of expanded sutures as a result of displacement.

Both of these methods of bone growth are used in different areas of the skull for its expansion in size and for its remodelling. Remodelling of growing bone maintains proportions within and between

71

bones. Sutural planes tend to be alined at right angles to the direction of movement of growing bones. The bony surfaces are orientated to slide with respect to one another, as the growing bones move apart. Displacement of bones is an important factor in the expansion of the craniofacial skeleton. The sliding characteristic of bone movement at angled sutural surfaces accommodates to the need for continued skeletal growth, and determines the direction of this growth. The basic suture type is the 'butt-end', or flat end-to-end type. Bevelling and serrations occur in sutures in response to functional demands outside of the sutures themselves. Sutural serrations are a gross manifestation of a form of trabecular growth responsive to tensions within the sutural tissues, set up in all probability by the rapidly expanding brain, eyeball, nasal septum, etc. (*Fig. 52*).

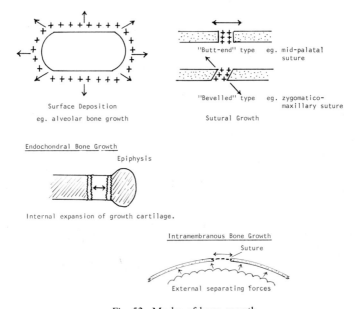

Fig. 52. Modes of bone growth.

Incremental growth at sutures does not take place only in the plane of the pre-existing curved bones. Differential rates of marginal and surface growth at the suture site allow the plane of growth to alter as the bone edges grow. Resorption of surface bone plays a significant role in this remodelling process. Differential apposition of bone leads to greater or lesser growth of one or other of the sutural bones, since each bony margin contributes independently of the other. In this manner both remodelling and growth can take place at suture sites. Advantage is taken of sutural growth potential in orthodontic treatment of skeletal deficiencies by forceful expansion techniques, as in intermaxillary expansion of narrow palates.

Sutural fusion, by ossification of the syndesmotic articulation, indicates cessation of growth at the suture concerned. There is great variability in the timing of sutural closures, making this phenomenon an unreliable criterion of age. Premature synostosis causes the cranium to be reduced in diameter at right angles to the fused suture, and abnormal compensatory growth occurs in other directions, resulting in malformation of the skull (e.g., *scaphocephaly*:wedge-shaped cranium; *acrocephaly* or *plagiocephaly*: pointed or twisted cranium).

SELECTED BIBLIOGRAPHY

BASSETT, C. A. L. (1966), 'Electro-mechanical Factors Regulating Bone Architecture', *3rd European Symposium on Calcified Tissues, Davos, Switzerland*. New York: Springer.

— — (1968), 'Biologic Significance of Piezo-electricity', *Calc. tiss. Res.*, **1**, 252.

— — (1972), 'A Biophysical Approach to Craniofacial Morphogenesis', *Acta morph. neerl.-scand.*, **10**, 71.

BOURNE, G. H. (Ed.) (1971), *The Biochemistry and Physiology of Bone*, 2nd ed., Vol. III, *Development and Growth*. New York: Academic Press.

CHAMAY, A., and TSCHANTZ, P. (1972), 'Mechanical Influences in Bone Remodeling. Experimental Research on Wolff's Law', *J. Biomech.*, **5**, 173.

DURKIN, J. F. (1972), 'Secondary Cartilage: a Misnomer?', *Am. J. Orthod.*, **62**, 15.

ENLOW, D. H. (1963), *Principles of Bone Remodeling*. Springfield, Ill.: Thomas.

— — (1968), 'Wolff's Law and the Factor of Architectonic Circumstance', *Am. J. Orthod.*, **54**, 803.

— — and HUNTER, W. S. (1966), 'A Differential Analysis of Sutural and Remodeling Growth in the Human Face', *Ibid.*, **52**, 823.

FRIEDENBERG, Z. B., HARLOW, M. C., HEPPENSTALL, R. B., and BRIGHTON, C. T. (1973), 'The Cellular Origin of Bioelectric Potentials in Bone', *Calc. tiss. Res.*, **13**, 53.

FROST, H. M. (1963), *Bone Remodelling Dynamics*. Springfield, Ill.: Thomas.

— — (1964), *The Laws of Bone Structure*. Springfield, Ill.: Thomas.

GLENISTER, T. W. (1976), 'An Embryological View of Cartilage', *J. Anat.*, **122**, 323.

HALL, B. K. (1978), *Developmental and Cellular Skeletal Biology*. New York: Academic Press.

HERMANSON, P. C. (1972), 'Alveolar Bone Remodeling Incident to Tooth Movement', *Angle Orthod.*, **42**, 107.

HWANG, W. S. (1978), 'Ultrastructure of Human Foetal and Neonatal Hyaline Cartilage', *J. Path.*, **126**, 209.

KOSKI, K. (1968), 'Cranial Growth Centres: Facts or Fallacies?', *Am. J. Orthod.*, **54**, 566.

MCKUSICK, V. A., and SCOTT, C. I. (1971), 'A Nomenclature for Constitutional Disorders of Bone', *J. Bone Jt Surg.*, **53A**, 978.

O'RAHILLY, R., and GARDNER, E. (1972), 'The Initial Appearance of Ossification in Staged Human Embryos', *Am. J. Anat.*, **134**, 291.

PRITCHARD, J. J. (1972), 'The Control or Trigger Mechanism Induced by Mechanical Forces which Causes Responses of Mesenchymal Cells in General and Bone Apposition and Resorption in Particular', *Acta morph. neerl.-scand.*, **10**, 63.

SARNAT, B. G. (1971), 'Clinical and Experimental Considerations in Facial Bone Biology: Growth, Remodelling and Repair', *J. Am. dent. Ass.* **82**, 876.

STOREY, E. (1972), 'Growth and Remodelling of Bone and Bones', *Am. J. Orthod.*, **62**, 142.

TANAKA, O. (1976), 'Time of the Appearance of Cartilage Centers in Human Embryos with Special Reference to its Individual Difference', *Okajimas Folia Anat. Jap.*, **53**, 173.

SECTION II

CRANIOFACIAL DEVELOPMENT

In the closest union there is still some separate existence of component parts; in the most complete separation there is still a reminiscence of union.

THE NOTEBOOKS OF SAMUEL BUTLER

INTRODUCTION

DEVELOPMENT of the skull, comprised of both the cranium and mandible, is a blend of the morphogenesis and growth of three main skull entities (*Fig. 53*). These skull entities are comprised of the following components:

1. *The Neurocranium*

The Vault of the Skull or Calvaria: phylogenetically of recent origin to cover the newly expanded brain, it is formed from intramembranous bone, and is known as the *desmocranium* (*desmos:* membrane).

The Cranial Base: derived from the phylogenetically ancient cranial floor with which are associated the capsular investments of the nasal and auditory sense organs; formed from endochondral bone, its cartilaginous precursor is known as the *chondrocranium* (*chondros:* cartilage).

2. *The Face*

The Orognathofacial Complex: derived from modifications of the phylogenetically ancient branchial arch structures; formed from intramembranous bone, it is also known as the *splanchnocranium* (*splanchnos:* viscus) or *viscerocranium* (viscus: an organ); this complex forms the oromasticatory musculature and jaw bones.

3. *The Masticatory Apparatus*

The Dentition: derived phylogenetically from ectodermal placoid scales, which is reflected in the embryological development of the teeth from oral ectoderm (dental lamina).

The cranial base is, to some extent, shared by both the neurocranial and the facial elements. The masticatory apparatus is composed of both facial and dental elements. The total skull is thus a mosaic of individual components, each of which enlarges during growth in the proper amount and direction to attain and maintain the stability of the whole.

Each of the three main craniofacial entities exhibits different characteristics of growth, development, maturation, and function. Yet each of the units is so integrated with the other that co-ordination of growth is required for normal development to occur. Failure of correlation of the various localized growth patterns, or aberration of inception, or growth, of an individual component, results in distorted craniofacial relationships, and is a factor in the development of dental malocclusion. While the neurocranium and face both have mixed intramembranous and endochondral types of bone formation, the bony elements of the masticatory apparatus are predominantly of intramembranous origin. The dental tissues have an ectodermal origin for their enamel and a neural crest origin for much of the mesenchyme that forms the dentine, pulp, cementum and periodontal ligament.

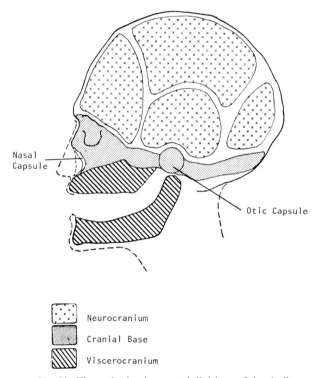

Nasal Capsule

Otic Capsule

☒ Neurocranium

▨ Cranial Base

▧ Viscerocranium

Fig. 53. The main developmental divisions of the skull.

It is of interest that the historically more recent developments in the mammalian skull, namely the membrane bones of the jaws and facial skeleton (splanchnocranium), are more susceptible to developmental anomalies than are the older cartilaginous parts of the skull. Developmental defects of the face and jaws are relatively common, whereas congenital defects of the skull base and of the nasal and otic (auditory) capsules are relatively rare. During postnatal growth of congenital craniofacial defects, three general patterns of development have been observed. Cases of hypoplastic defects may

77

demonstrate substantial improvement with 'catch-up' growth minimizing the defect. Alternatively, the defective pattern of growth is maintained throughout infancy or childhood so that the deformity is retained to the same degree in the adult as in the infant. The third pattern is one in which the developmental derangement worsens with age, so that the severity of the deformity is greater in the adult than in the child.

The differentiation of the chondrocranium appears to be strongly genetically determined, and subject to minimal environmental influence. The growth of the desmocranium and splanchnocranium, on the other hand, appears to be subject to minimal genetic determination, while the influence of local environmental factors is strong.

For descriptive convenience, details of the growth and development of the head have been subdivided into the following components:

The calvaria
The cranial base
The facial skeleton
The palate
The paranasal sinuses
The mandible
The temporomandibular joint
Skull growth: sutures and cephalometrics
The tongue and tonsils
The salivary glands
Muscle development
The special sense organs
The dentition.

CHAPTER 7

THE CALVARIA

The Membranous Neurocranium (Desmocranium)

THE mesenchyme that gives rise to the vault of the neurocranium is first arranged as a capsular membrane around the developing brain. The membrane is composed of two layers, an inner *endomeninx*, of neural crest origin and an outer *ectomeninx*, of mesodermal origin (*Fig. 54*). The endomeninx forms the two leptomeningeal coverings of the brain—the pia mater and the arachnoid. The ectomeninx differentiates into the inner dura mater covering the brain, which remains unossified, and an outer superficial membrane with chondrogenic and osteogenic properties. Osteogenesis of the ectomeninx occurs as intramembranous bone formation over the dome of the brain, forming the skull vault or calvaria, while the ectomeninx forming the floor of the brain chondrifies as the chondrocranium that later ossifies endochondrally (*see* Chapter 8).

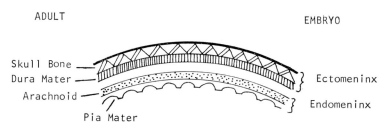

Fig. 54. The embryonic and adult components of the desmocranium.

Despite their divergent fates, the two layers of the ectomeninx remain in close apposition, except in regions where the venous sinuses develop. The dura mater and its septa, the falces cerebri and cerebelli and the tentorium cerebelli, show distinctly organized fibre bundles closely related and strongly attached to the sutural systems that later develop in the vault. The adult form of the neurocranium is the end-result of the preferential direction of the forces set up by the growth of the brain along these dural fibre systems.

In the somite period embryo, the neural tube's covering dura mater and the surface ectoderm are in contact in the area of the closing anterior neuropore of the developing brain. Transient maintenance

79

of this contact during development causes a dural projection that, consequent to ventral bending of the rostrum, extends into the future frontonasal suture area. Later, as the nasal capsules (p. 89) surround the dural projection, the resulting midline canal forms the basis of the *foramen caecum* in the subsequently developed ethmoid-frontal bone junctional region. The dural projection and frontonasal area skin normally separate by withdrawal of the dural projection, allowing for sealing of the canal and consequent closing of the foramen caecum (hence 'blind foramen'). Failure of closure of the foramen caecum allows an abnormal pathway for neural tissue to herniate into the nasal region (*see* p. 111).

Ossification of the intramembranous calvarial bones depends upon the presence of the brain, for in its absence (anencephaly) no bony calvaria forms. Several primary and secondary ossification centres develop in the outer layer of the ectomeninx to form individual bones. A pair of *frontal bones* appears from single primary ossification centres forming in the region of each superciliary arch at the 8th week i.u. Three pairs of secondary centres appear later—in the zygomatic processes, nasal spine and trochlear fossae. Fusion between all these centres is complete at 6–7 months i.u. At birth the frontal bones are separated by the frontal (metopic) suture. Synostotic fusion of the suture usually commences about the second year uniting the frontal bones into a single bone by 7 years of age.*

The two *parietal bones* arise from two primary ossification centres for each bone that appear at the parietal eminence in the 8th week i.u. and fuse soon after. Delayed ossification in the region of the parietal foramina may result in the presence of a sagittal fontanelle at birth.

The supranuchal *squamous portion of the occipital bone* (above the superior nuchal line) ossifies intramembranously from two centres, one on each side, appearing in the 8th week i.u. The rest of the occipital bone ossifies endochondrally (*see* p. 92).

The *squamous portion of the temporal bone*† ossifies intramembranously from a single centre appearing at the root of the zygoma at the 8th week i.u. The *tympanic-ring of the temporal bone* ossifies intramembranously from one centre appearing in the 3rd month i.u. in the lateral wall of the tympanum. Fusion of the two membranous bone portions of the temporal bone occurs at birth. The rest of the temporal bone ossifies endochondrally (*see* p. 93).

---

*The frontal (metopic) suture persists into adulthood in about 15 per cent of skulls.

†The squamous temporal bone is independent of brain induction and is present in anencephaly.

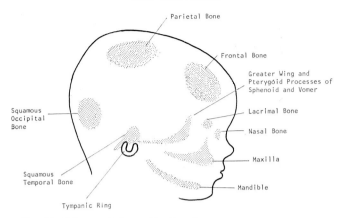

Parietal Bone

Frontal Bone

Greater Wing and
Pterygóid Processes of
Sphenoid and Vomer

Squamous
Occipital
Bone

Lacrimal Bone

Nasal Bone

Maxilla

Squamous
Temporal Bone

Mandible

Tympanic Ring

Fig. 55. Schema of the ossification sites of the intramembranous bones of the skull.

Should any unusual ossification centres develop between individual calvarial bones, their independent existence is recognized as small *sutural* or *Wormian bones.** The earliest centres of ossification first appear during the 7th and 8th weeks i.u., but ossification is not completed until well after birth (*Fig. 55*). The mesenchyme between the bones develops fibres to form syndesmotic articulations. The membranous mesenchyme covering the bones forms the periosteum. At birth, the individual calvarial bones are separated by sutures of variable width and by fontanelles. Six of these fontanelles are identified as the anterior, posterior, posterolateral, and anterolateral, in relation to the corners of the two parietal bones (*Fig. 56*). The presence of these flexible membranous junctions between the calvarial bones allows narrowing of the sutures and fontanelles and overriding of these bones to occur when compressed during birth (*Fig. 57*). The head may appear distorted for several days after birth.

Postnatal bone growth results in narrowing of the width of the sutures and elimination of the fontanelles. The anterolateral fontanelles† close 3 months after birth; the posterolateral fontanelles are closed at the end of the first year; the posterior fontanelle closes 2 months after birth, and the anterior fontanelle during the

---

*Wormian bones occur most frequently along the lambdoid suture, where they form interparietal bones, sometimes called 'Inca bones', because of their frequent appearance in Inca people. Development of these ossicles may have a genetic component, but as hydrocephalic crania almost always exhibit wormian bones, deforming stress appears to be a contributing factor.

†The site of the anterolateral fontanelle corresponds with pterion in the adult skull; the site of the posterolateral fontanelle corresponds with asterion.

second year. The median frontal suture is usually obliterated between 6 and 8 years of age. This extension of ossification of the calvarial bones continues throughout life. The syndesmosal sutures between the neurocranial bones fuse into synostoses with advancing years, uniting the individual calvarial bones into a single component

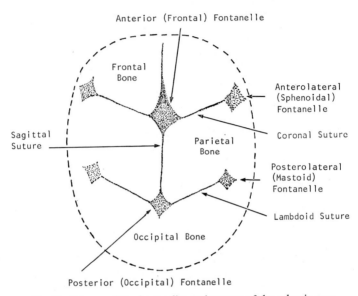

Fig. 56. Schema of the fontanelles and sutures of the calvaria seen from above.

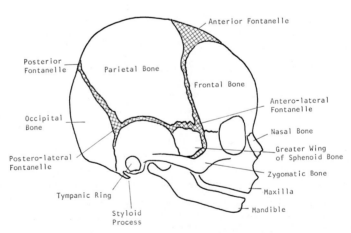

Fig. 57. The bones of the neonatal skull and the intervening sutures and fontanelles.

82

in old age. In the fetus, the intramembranous neurocranial bones are moulded into large, slightly curved 'plates' over the expanding brain which they cover. The precocious development of the brain determines the early predominance of the neurocranium over the facial and masticatory portions of the skull. While the brain, and consequently the neurocranial bone vault, develop very rapidly very early, they also slow down and cease growing at an earlier age than do the facial and masticatory elements of the skull. The predominance of the neurocranium over the face is greatest in the early fetus, reducing to an 8 to 1 proportion at birth, 6 to 1 in the second year, 4 to 1 in the fifth year and a 2–2½ to 1 proportion in the adult.

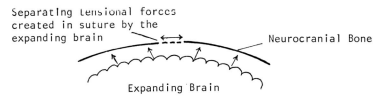

Fig. 58. Schematic section through skull and brain to demonstrate the action of 'functional matrix' growth forces.

At birth, the neurocranium has achieved 25 per cent of its ultimate growth, completing 50 per cent at age 6 months and 75 per cent at 2 years. While 95 per cent of neurocranial growth has been completed by the tenth year of age, the facial skeleton has achieved only 65 per cent of its total growth by that age. In postnatal life the neurocranium increases 4–5 times in volume, while the facial portion increases some 8–10 times its volume at birth.

The ultimate shape and size of the cranial vault are primarily dependent upon the internal pressures exerted on the inner table of the neurocranial bones. The expanding brain exerts separating tensional forces upon the bone sutures, thereby secondarily stimulating compensatory sutural bone growth (*Fig. 58*). The brain acts in this context as a 'functional matrix' in determining the extent of neurocranial bone growth. The circumference of the head, because it is related to intracranial volume, is a valuable indicator of brain growth.* The precocious early development of the brain is reflected in the rapidly enlarging circumference of the head, which nearly doubles from an average of 18 cm. at the mid-gestational period

---

*Between birth and adulthood, brain size increases about 3½ times, from approximately 400 c.c. to 1300–1400 c.c. The early rapid expansion of the brain poses problems for the already established cerebral blood vessels that, by being stretched, weakens their walls, predisposing to aneurysm formation in later life.

(4·5 months) to an average of 33 cm. (approx. 13 in.) at birth. This rapid increase of head circumference continues during the first year to reach an average of 46 cm. Head circumference growth slows down thereafter to reach 49 cm. at two years, and only 50 cm. at three years. The increase between three years and adulthood is only about 6 cm.

Growth of the calvarial bones is a combination of: (1) sutural growth, (2) surface apposition and resorption (remodelling), and (3) outward displacement caused by the expanding brain. The proportions between the different growth mechanisms vary. Accretion to the calvarial bones is predominantly sutural until about the fourth year of life, after which surface apposition becomes increasingly important. Remodelling of the curved bony plates allows for their flattening out to accommodate the increasing surface area of the growing brain. The flattening of the early high curvature of the calvarial bones is achieved by a combination of endocranial erosion and ectocranial deposition, in addition to which there is ectocranial resorption from certain areas of maximal curvature, such as the frontal and parietal eminences.

The bones of the newborn calvaria are unilaminar and lack diploë. From about four years of age, lamellar compaction of cancellous trabeculae form the inner and outer tables of the cranial bones. The tables become continuously more distinct into adulthood. While the behaviour of the inner table is related primarily to the brain and intracranial pressures, the outer table is more responsive to extracranial muscular forces. However, the two cortical plates are not completely independent. The thickening of the frontal bone in the midline at glabella results from the invasion of the frontal sinus between the cortical plates, but only the external plate is remodelled, as the internal plate becomes stable at 6–7 years of age. Thus, only the inner aspect of the frontal bone can be used as a stable (X-ray) reference point for growth studies from age 7 years onwards. Growth of the external plate during childhood produces the superciliary arches, mastoid processes, external occipital protuberance and the temporal and nuchal lines that are absent from the neonatal skull. The bones of the calvaria continue to increase slowly in thickness even after completion of their general growth.

When intracranial pressures become excessive, as occurs in the pathological condition of hydrocephalus, both plates of the bones of the calvaria become thinned and grossly expanded. Conversely, the reduced functional matrix force of the brain in microcephalics results in a small calvaria. Normal forces acting on the outer table of bone alone tend to influence the superstructure of the cranium only, and not the intracranial form. The pull of muscles would account to some degree for the development of the mastoid process, the lateral pterygoid plate, the temporal and nuchal lines in the cranium, the coronoid process and the ramus–body angle of the mandible. In the face, the buttressing resistance to masticatory forces produces the supraorbital processes. These superstructural bony projections add to the dimension of the cranium, but are unrelated to the intracranial capacity. Abnormal external forces applied during development can distort cranial morphology, but, strangely enough, not cranial capacity, as is evident by the bizarre shapes of skulls produced by pressure devices on children's skulls in some primitive American Indian societies (*Fig. 59*).

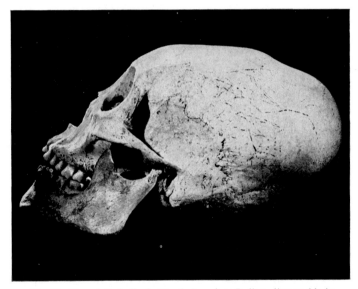

Fig. 59. The adult skull of a North American Indian, distorted in its growth into an anteroposterior elongation by the application of head-boards during infancy.

The calvaria is particularly susceptible to a number of congenital defects ranging from chromosomal to hormonal in their aetiology. The time of closure of the sutures is altered in many of these afflictions, leading to variable distortions of skull shape. In such widely different conditions as cretinism, progeria, trisomy 21, and cleidocranial dysostosis, there is a delayed midline ossification of the frontal (metopic) and sagittal sutures of the calvaria, associated with which the anterior fontanelle may remain open into adult life. The resulting brachycephalic skull in these conditions displays a 'bossed' forehead of highly curved frontal and parietal bones together with hypertelorism that obscures the generally reduced size of the brain case.

Premature fusion of the coronal suture characterizes cases of acrocephalosyndactyly (Apert's syndrome), and early synostosis of the coronal, sagittal, and lambdoid sutures occurs in craniofacial dysostosis (Crouzon's syndrome). The inability of the calvaria to grow normally in both of these conditions leads to skull distortion known as acrocephaly, oxycephaly, or turricephaly, all characterized by peaking of the vault of the skull. These skull anomalies worsen during the growth period of the child.

SELECTED BIBLIOGRAPHY

EL-NAJJAR, M. Y., and DAWSON, G. L. (1977), 'The Effect of Artificial Cranial Deformation on the Incidence of Wormian Bones in the Lambdoidal Suture', *Am. J. Phys. Anthrop.*, **46**, 155.

ENLOW, D. H., KURODA, T., and LEWIS, A. B. (1971), 'The Morphological and Morphogenetic Basis for Craniofacial Form and Pattern', *Angle Orth.*, **41**, 161.

FERGUSON, M. W. J. (1980), 'Turricephaly', *Int. J. Oral Surg.*, **9**, 343.

GRUBE, D., and REINBACH, W. (1976), 'Das Cranium eines menschlichen Embryo von 80 mm Sch.-St.-Länge', *Anat. Embryol.*, **149**, 183.

KISLING, E. (1966), *Cranial Morphology in Down's Syndrome*. Copenhagen: Munksgaard.

LAVELLE, C. L. B. (1974), 'An Analysis of Foetal Craniofacial Growth', *Ann. hum. Biol.*, **1**, 269.

MALINOWSKI, A. (1970), 'The Length, Width, and Cranial Index in Human Fetuses', *Folia Morph.*, **29**, 438.

MEREDITH, H. V. (1971), 'Human Head Circumference from Birth to Early Adulthood: Racial, Regional and Sex Comparisons', *Growth*, **35**, 233.

MOYERS, R. E., and KROGMAN, W. M. (ed.) (1971), *Cranio-facial Growth in Man*. Oxford: Pergamon.

NELLHAUS, G. (1968), 'Head Circumference from Birth to Eighteen Years: Practical Composite International and Interracial Graphs', *Pediatrics*, **41**, Part I, 106.

SMITH, G. F., and BERG, J. M. (1976), *Down's Anomaly* (2nd ed.) pp. 43–50. Edinburgh: Churchill Livingstone.

SRIVASTAVA, H. C. (1977), 'Development of Ossification Centres in the Squamous Portion of the Occipital Bone in Man', *J. Anat.*, **124**, 643.

CHAPTER 8

THE CRANIAL BASE

The Chondrocranium

DURING the 4th week, mesenchyme derived from the primitive streak and neural crest condenses between the developing brain and foregut to form the basal portion of the ectomeningeal capsule. This condensation betokens the earliest evidence of skull formation. Even then, development of the skull starts comparatively late, after the primordia of many of the other cranial structures, such as the brain, cranial nerves, the eyes, and the blood-vessels have already developed. During the late somite period the occipital sclerotomal mesenchyme concentrates around the notochord underlying the developing hindbrain. From this region the mesenchymal concentration extends cephalically, forming a floor for the developing brain. Conversion of the ectomeninx mesenchyme into cartilage* constitutes the beginning of the chondrocranium that commences from the 40th day i.u. onwards.

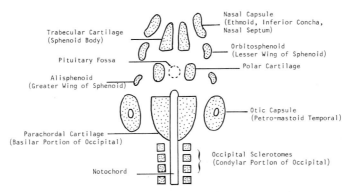

Fig. 60. The primordial cartilages of the chondrocranium.

Chondrification centres forming around the cranial end of the notochord are appropriately called the *parachordal cartilages* (*Fig. 60*). From the parachordal cartilages a caudal extension of chondrification incorporates the fused sclerotomes arising from the four occipital somites surrounding the neural tube. The sclerotome

---

*The formation of the cartilages of the chondrocranium is dependent upon the presence of the brain and other neural structures.

87

cartilage forms the boundaries of the foramen magnum, providing the anlagen for the basilar and condylar parts of the occipital bone.

The cranial end of the notochord coincides with the level of the oropharyngeal membrane that closes off the stomodeum. Just cranial to the oropharyngeal membrane, the hypophyseal (Rathke's) pouch, arising from the stomodeum, gives rise to the anterior lobe of the pituitary gland (adenohypophysis) which accordingly lies immediately cranial to the termination of the notochord (*Fig. 61*). In this region two *hypophyseal* (*postsphenoid*) *cartilages* develop on either side of the hypophyseal stem and fuse to form the *basisphenoid* (*postsphenoid*) cartilage containing the hypophysis, and will later give rise to the sella turcica and posterior part of the body of the sphenoid bone.

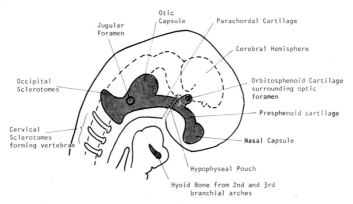

Fig. 61. Schematic sagittal section through the head of an embryo of the late embryonic period (7th week). Fused chondrocranial cartilages form the basal plate.

Cranial to the pituitary gland, two *presphenoid* (*trabecular*) cartilages fuse together to form the precursor to the presphenoid bone that will form the anterior part of the body of the sphenoid bone. Laterally, the chondrification centres of the *orbitosphenoid* (lesser wing) and *alisphenoid* (greater wing) contribute wings to the sphenoid bone. Most anteriorly, the fused presphenoid cartilages become a vertical cartilaginous plate within the nasal septum called the *mesethmoid cartilage*. The mesethmoid cartilage ossifies at birth into the *perpendicular plate of the ethmoid bone*, its upper edge forming the *crista galli* that separates the olfactory bulbs.

The capsules surrounding the nasal and otic (vestibulocochlear) sense organs chondrify and fuse to the cartilages of the cranial base.

The *nasal capsules*★ chondrify in the 2nd month i.u. to form a box of cartilage with a roof and lateral walls divided by a median cartilage septum (*Fig. 62*). Ossification centres in the lateral walls of the capsule form the *lateral masses* (*labyrinths*) of the *ethmoid* and the *inferior nasal concha* bones.

The median nasal septum remains cartilaginous except postero-inferiorly, where in the membrane on each side of the septum, intra-membranous ossification centres form the initially paired *vomer* bone, its two halves uniting below before birth, but containing intervening nasal septal cartilage until puberty. Appositional bone growth postnatally on the posterosuperior margins of the vomer contribute to nasal septal growth and indirectly to the downward and forward growth of the face (*Fig. 63*).

The chondrified nasal capsules form the *cartilages of the nostrils* and the nasal septal cartilage. In the fetus, the septal cartilage inter-venes between the cranial base above and the 'premaxilla', vomer and palatal processes of the maxilla below.† The nasal septal cartilage is equivocally believed, by its growth, to play a role in the downward and forward growth of the midface (acting as a 'functional matrix'). (*See* p. 106.)

The *otic capsules* chondrify and fuse with the parachordal cartilages to ossify later as the mastoid and petrous portions of the temporal bones. The optic capsule does not chondrify in the human subject.

The initially separate centres of cranial base chondrification fuse into a single, irregular, and greatly perforated *basal plate*. The early establishment of the blood-vessels, cranial nerves, and spinal cord between the developing brain and its extracranial contacts, prior to chondrification, determines the presence of the numerous perfora-tions (foramina) in the cartilage basal plate, and in the subsequent osseous cranial floor (*Fig. 64*).

The ossifying chondrocranium meets the ossifying desmocranium to form the neurocranium. The developing brain lies in the shallow groove formed by the chondrocranium. The deep central hypo-physeal fossa is bounded by the presphenoid cartilage of the tuber-culum sellae anteriorly and the postsphenoid cartilage of the dorsum sellae posteriorly.

★The nasal capsule and nasal septum have been postulated to arise from pre-chordal (pre-otic) sclerotomes; the myotomes of these prechordal somites are presumed to give rise to the extrinsic eye muscles.

Contrariwise, experimental studies indicate the nasal septum and posterior nasal walls represents a premandibular visceral arch cartilage of neural crest origin. The roof and sidewalls of the nasal capsule, while also of ectomesen-chymal origin, have the nasal placodes as a source of cartilage.

†Postnatally the septal cartilage may act as a strut to resist the compressive forces of incision, transferring these forces from the incisor region to the sphenoid bone.

The fibres of the olfactory nerve (I) determine the perforations of the cribriform plate of the ethmoid bone. Extensions of the orbito-sphenoid cartilage around the optic nerve (II) and ophthalmic artery, when fusing with the cranial part of the basal plate, form the *optic foramen*. The initial space between the orbitosphenoid and alisphenoid cartilages is retained by the passage of the oculomotor (III), trochlear (IV), ophthalmic (V^1) and abducens (VI) nerves and the ophthalmic veins as the *superior orbital fissure*. The junction of

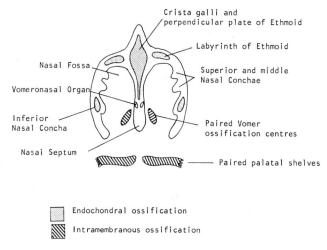

Fig. 62. Schema of coronal section of nasal capsules and ossification centres.

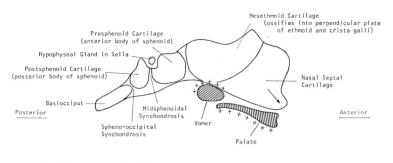

Fig. 63. The median sagittal cartilages of the fetal chondrocranium.

90

the alisphenoid (greater wing) and polar (body) cartilages of the sphenoid bone is interrupted by the passages of the maxillary nerve (V²) to create the *foramen rotundum*, of the mandibular nerve (V³) to create the *foramen ovale*, and of the middle meningeal artery to form the *foramen spinosum*. Persistence of the cartilage between the ossification sites of the alisphenoid and the otic capsule accounts for the existence of the *foramen lacerum*. Ossification around the internal carotid artery accounts for its canal, interposed at the junctional site of the alisphenoid and polar cartilages and otic capsule. The passage of the facial (VII) and vestibulocochlear (VIII) nerves through the otic capsule ensures the existence of the *internal acoustic meatus*. The glossopharyngeal (IX), vagus (X), and spinal accessory (XI) nerves and the internal jugular vein passing between the otic capsule and the parachordal cartilage account for the large *jugular foramen*. The hypoglossal nerve (XII) passing between the occipital sclerotomes accounts for the *hypoglossal* or *anterior condylar canal*.

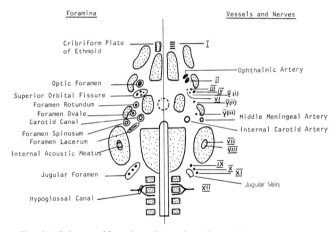

Fig. 64. Schema of location of vessels and cranial nerves numbered I–XII, (*right*) and foramina (*left*) in the chondrocranial base.

Chondrocranial Ossification

Approximately 110 ossification centres appear in the embryonic human skull. Many of these centres fuse to produce 45 separate bones in the neonatal skull. In the young adult, 32 separate skull bones are recognized.

Centres of ossification within the basal plate, commencing with the basioccipital in the 10th week i.u. lay the basis for the endochondral bone portions of the occipital, sphenoid and temporal bones (all of which also have intramembranous bone components) and for the wholly endochondral ethmoid and inferior nasal concha bones (*Fig. 65*).

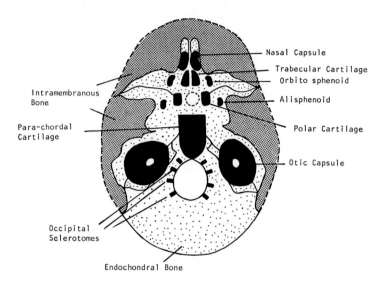

Fig. 65. Schema of adult cranial base indicating sites of primordial cartilages of chondrocranium (*in black*) and extent of endochondral (*light stipple*) and intramembranous (*heavy stipple*) ossification.

The Occipital Bone

Seven ossification centres (two intramembranous, five endochondral) appear for the occipital bone. The supranuchal squamous part ossifies intramembranously from a pair of ossification centres appearing in the 8th week i.u. Below the superior nuchal line, the rest of the squamous portion ossifies endochondrally from two centres, one on each side, that appear at the 10th week i.u. By the 12th week, all four squamous centres have fused. The basilar part ossifies endochondrally from a single median centre appearing at the 11th week i.u. This part forms the anterior boundary of the foramen magnum and small anterior portions of the occipital condyles. A pair of condylar endochondral centres appears at 12 weeks i.u. in the occipital sclerotome cartilages, forming the lateral boundaries of the foramen magnum and the major posterior

92

portions of the occipital condyles around the hypoglossal canals. A synchondrosis between the two portions of the occipital condyles exists in the neonatal skull and persists until the age of 3 or 4 years, when ossification of this synchondrosis commences, and is completed by age 7 years. By this age, the squamous, condylar and basilar portions of the occipital have united into a single bone.

During postnatal life, the endocranial surfaces of the occipital bone are predominantly resorptive, and the ectocranial surfaces depository, producing a downward displacement of the floor of the posterior cranial fossa.

The Temporal Bone

This complex bone of four parts ossifies in membrane and cartilage from 11 centres. The *squamous* portion ossifies intramembranously from a single centre appearing in the 8th week i.u. The *tympanic ring*, also formed of intramembranous bone, ossifies from four centres starting in the 3rd month i.u. The *petromastoid* temporal ossifies endochondrally in the otic capsule from four centres that appear about the 5th month i.u. and fuse about the 6th month i.u. The otic capsule encloses the developing middle and inner ears. The inner ear reaches adult size by 18 weeks, before ossification* of the capsule commences. The *styloid process* ossifies in the cartilage of the hyoid (second) branchial arch (*see* p. 57) from two centres, the upper centre appearing just before birth and the lower after birth.

At birth, the tympanic ring is fused with the squamous temporal and later grows laterally to form the *tympanic plate*. During the first postnatal year, the petromastoid portion fuses with the squamous portion and the proximal part of the styloid process. The distal part of the styloid process unites with the proximal at about puberty. Growth of the mastoid process occurs mostly after the second year of life, when it is invaded by extensions of the tympanic antrum to form mastoid air cells.

The Ethmoid Bone (Fig. 62, p. 90)

This wholly endochondral bone that forms the median floor of the anterior cranial fossa, and parts of the roof, lateral walls and median septum of the nasal cavity ossifies from three centres—a single median centre in the mesethmoid cartilage derived from the nasal septum, forming the perpendicular plate and crista galli appearing just before birth, and one lateral centre for each labyrinth, appearing in the nasal capsular cartilages at the 4th month i.u. At two years

*The fetal-type of bone laid down in the otic capsule is uniquely retained throughout life, and is not replaced as elsewhere by haversian bone. The ossified otic capsule becomes embedded in the petrous portion of the temporal bone.

of age, the ethmoid perpendicular plate unites with the labyrinths by ossification of the cribriform plate to form a single ethmoid bone.

Resorption of the endocranial surface of the cribriform plates with deposition on the opposite nasal surface results in a downward movement of the anterior cranial floor. Widening of the cribriform plate takes place in relation to the increasing size of the nasal cavities.

Inferior Nasal Concha (*Fig. 62*, p. 90)

This endochondral bone ossifies in the cartilage of the lateral part of the nasal capsule from a single centre that appears in the 5th month i.u.

The Sphenoid Bone

Ossification of the sphenoid bone is extraordinarily complex. Up to 15 separate ossification centres may appear in the sphenoid anlagen that are of both intramembranous and endochondral origin. Two intramembranous ossification centres appear in the 8th week for part of the greater wing of the sphenoid and for the lateral pterygoid plate.

The medial pterygoid plate ossifies endochondrally from a secondary cartilage located in its hamular process. Endochondral ossification centres appear for the lesser wing of the sphenoid (in the orbitosphenoid cartilage), for a portion of the greater wing of the sphenoid (in the alisphenoid cartilage) and for anterior (presphenoid) and posterior (postsphenoid) parts of the sphenoid body. The presphenoid, arising from five ossification centres (two paired and a median unpaired) appearing in the presphenoid and nasal septal cartilages in the 4th month i.u. forms the sphenoid body anterior to the tuberculum sellae. The postsphenoid, arising from four ossification centres (two in each hypophyseal cartilage) forms the sella turcica, dorsum sellae and basisphenoid.

The four ossification centres of the postsphenoid appear early in the 4th month i.u. and coalesce late in the 4th month. This coalescence of ossification centres obliterates the pharyngohypophyseal track* of Rathke's pouch that forms the adenohypophysis.

A midsphenoidal synchondrosis between the pre- and postsphenoid fuses shortly before birth.† The bases of the pterygoid

---

*A craniophyaryngeal canal between the floor of the sella turcica and the inferior surface of the sphenoid body persists in 0·4 per cent of postnatal skulls, forming the basis of craniopharyngeal tumours.

†In most mammals other than man, the midsphenoidal synchondrosis remains unfused permanently, or fuses late in the postnatal growth period.

plates fuse with the postsphenoid soon after birth, the fusing bone surrounding the nerve of the pterygoid canal.

The chondrocranium is important as a junction between the neurocranial and facial skeletons, being shared by both. The cranial base is relatively stable during growth compared with the calvaria and face, providing some basis against which the growth of the latter skull elements can be compared. The extremely rapid growth of the neurocranium and particularly of the calvaria contrasts with the slower but more prolonged growth of the facial skeleton. The chondrocranial base of the newborn skull is small compared to the calvarial desmocranial part that extends beyond the base laterally and posteriorly. The relative stability of the chondrocranium maintains the early-established relationships of the blood-vessels, cranial nerves, and spinal cord running through it from their sources to their destinations.

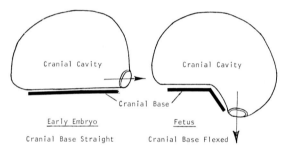

Fig. 66. Diagrammatic representation of the flexure of the cranial base, altering the direction of the foramen magnum from the horizontal to the vertical (arrows).

During the embryonic and early fetal periods, the cranial base becomes flexed in the region between the pituitary fossa and the spheno-occipital junction, so that the developing face becomes tucked in under the cranium. The ventral surface of the developing brain-stem similarly becomes flexed at the site of the dorsum sellae of the pituitary fossa with the result that the spinal cord alters its original posterior relationship to the rest of the brain to an inferior one. Concomitantly, the exit of the spinal cord from the skull—the foramen magnum—changes from its posteriorly directed location in the skull to a vertical downward direction near the middle of the inferior surface of the skull. This cranial base flexure effectively enlarges the neurocranial capacity (*Fig. 66*). The downwardly directed foramen magnum is related to an upright (bipedal) posture, and to an increased cranial capacity, both of which are features of

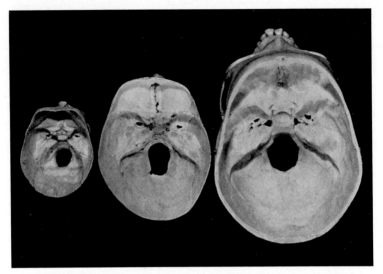

Fig. 67. The cranial bases of a neonate (*left*), a one-year-old child (*centre*) and an adult (*right*) demonstrating the relatively small amount of growth in the brain-stem area (sella turcica, clivus and foramen magnum) compared to the enormous expansion of the surrounding parts. Note also the thickening of the calvarial bones from infancy to adulthood, and the beginning of development of diploë in the one-year-old skull.

man. A further consequence of the cranial flexure,* and also a peculiarly hominid characteristic, is the predominantly downward, rather than forward, displacement of the face during its growth from the cranial base.

The growth of the cranial base is highly uneven in keeping with the highly irregular shape it develops to accommodate the undulating ventral surface of the brain. The uneven growth of the different portions of the brain is reflected in the related parts of the cranial base adapting as compartments or cranial fossae. The anterior and posterior parts of the cranial base grow at different rates.

*Flexion of the chondrocranial base in the 10 week old fetus, before ossification occurs, produces an angle of 65° between the anterior and posterior parts of the chondrocranium. This angle subsequently opens out to a less acute angle at birth.

Down's syndrome and Turner's syndrome subjects display a greater than normal flexure of the cranial base. Achondroplasia and chondrodystrophia subjects show increased angulation of the cranial base. This can be ascribed to a loss of the flattening effect usually produced by late growth at the spheno-occipital synchondrosis. Anencephalics retain the acute cranial base flexure found in the early fetus, suggesting brain growth contributes to flattening of the cranial base.

Between the 10th and 40th weeks i.u., the anterior cranial base increases its length and width sevenfold, while in the same period, the posterior cranial base grows fivefold. The central ventral axis of the brain (the brain-stem) is of conservative growth, and is related to the body of the sphenoid and basioccipital bones, that, by their slow growth, provide a comparatively stable base. Laterally, cranially, and caudal to this base, the anterior, middle and posterior fossae of the cranial floor, related to the frontal and temporal lobes of the cerebrum, and to the cerebellum respectively, expand enormously in keeping with the exuberant efflorescence of these parts of the brain (*Figs. 67, 68*).

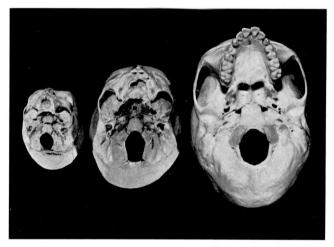

Fig. 68. The skull bases of a neonate (*left*), a one-year-old child (*centre*) and an adult (*right*) demonstrating the extent of anterior (facial) growth. In the neonate skull, note the presence of the posterolateral fontanelles and the presence of the four parts (basi-occiput, condylar and squamous parts) of the occipital bone before they fuse into a single bone around the foramen magnum. Note also the flat occipital condyles and absent articular tubercles and mastoid processes in the newborn skull.

Expansion of the cranial base takes place as a result of: (1) growth of the cartilage remnants of the chondrocranium that persist between the bones, and (2) expansive forces emanating from the growing brain (a capsular functional matrix) displacing the bones at the suture lines (*Fig. 69*). By their interstitial growth, the interposed cartilages, known as *synchondroses*, can separate the adjacent bones as appositional bone growth adds to their sutural edges. Thus,

97

growth of the bones within the ventral midline, the cribriform plate of the ethmoid, the pre- and basisphenoid and the basi-occipital bones contribute to cranial base growth. The cartilages between these bones contribute variably to cranial elongation and lateral expansion. Growth in anteroposterior length of the anterior cranial fossa depends on growth at the sphenofrontal, fronto-ethmoidal and spheno-ethmoidal sutures. The last two sutures cease contributing to sagittal plane growth after the age of seven years. The internal surfaces of the frontal bone and cribriform plate cease remodelling at about 4 years of age, thereby becoming 'stable' from about 6–7 years of age. Further growth of the anterior cranial base (anterior to the foramen caecum) is associated with expansion of the developing frontal air sinuses.

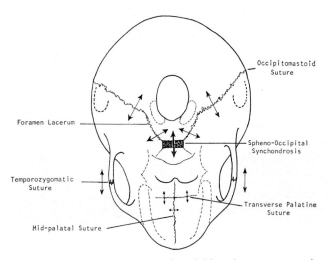

Fig. 69. Directions of growth of cranial base bones at suture sites, accounting for multi-directional expansion of the cranial base.

Postnatal growth activity in the spheno-occipital synchondrosis★ is the major contributor to growth of the cranial base, as it persists into early adulthood. This prolonged growth period allows for continued posterior expansion of the maxilla to accommodate later erupting molar teeth, and provides space for the growing naso-pharynx. The spheno-occipital synchondrosis is the last of the synchondroses to fuse, beginning on its cerebral surface at 12–13

★Prenatally, this synchondrosis is not a major growth site. Postnatally, greater bone deposition occurs on the occipital than on the sphenoidal side of the synchondrosis that proliferates interstitially in its midzone.

years in girls, and 14–15 years in boys, and completing ossification of the external aspect by 20 years of age.*

In addition to proliferative synchondrosal growth, the cranial base undergoes selective remodelling by resorption and deposition. The clivus, while resorbing on its cerebral surface, shows apposition on the nasopharyngeal (inferior) surface of the basi-occipital bone and the anterior margin of the foramen magnum, allowing lengthening of the clivus to occur after spheno-occipital synchondrosal closure. To maintain the size of the foramen magnum, resorption occurs at its posterior margin. The separate squamous, condylar and basilar parts of the occipital bone fuse together only after birth. The temporal bone is composed of its separate petrous, squamous, styloid and tympanic ring parts at birth, when their union commences. At birth, the temporal mandibular fossa is flat and lacks an articular tubercle. The occipital condyles are flat, and only become prominent during childhood.

During growth, marked resorption takes place in the floors of the cranial fossae, deepening these endocranial compartments. This deepening process is aided by the bodily displacement of the floors of the fossae as a result of sutural expansion of the lateral walls of the neurocranium. The increase in size of the sella turcica is due to remodelling of its inner contour. Although the anterior wall of the sella turcica is stable by 5–6 years of age, its posterior wall, and to a varying extent its floor, is resorbing until 16–17 years of age.†
Parts of the petrous portion of the temporal bone are exceptional to the generalized internal resorption of the cranial base in that some bone deposition may occur at this site.

Phylogenetically the oldest portion of the skull, the cranial base, is also the most conservative in expansive growth, of all the main elements that make up the skull. The differing areas of sutural accretion, surface deposition and resorption of bone, and the displacement, flexing, and readjustments of the bones of the cranial base to each other provide an extremely complicated pattern of overall growth. The dependence of the juxtaposed calvaria and facial skeleton upon the cranial base confers considerable significance upon its growth behaviour in determining the final shape and size of the cranium, and ultimately, the morphology of the entire skull,

---

*Continued growth of the inferior aspect of the synchondrosis, after fusion of its superior (cerebral) surface would result in an upward and backward displacement of the basi-occiput relative to the sphenoid, tending to flatten the spheno-occipital angle, and thus the cranial base. This tendency is counteracted by resorption internally of the clivus, thereby maintaining a fairly constant spheno-occipital angle during growth.

†Owing to the variable remodelling that occurs in the sella turcica, the reference point *sella* (the centre of the sella turcica) cannot be regarded as stable until well after puberty.

CRANIOFACIAL EMBRYOLOGY

including the occlusion of the dentition. Inadequate chondrocranial growth precludes sufficient allocation of space for full
eruption of the total dentition, particularly in the case of a diminished
maxilla, leading to impacted eruption of the last teeth to emerge,
viz. the third molars.

Afflictions of cartilage growth producing a reduced cranial base
result in a 'dished' deformity of the middle third of the facial skeleton,
and a rounding or 'brachycephalization' of the neurocranium. Such
diverse conditions as achondroplasia, cretinism, and Downs' syndrome (trisomy 21) all produce a similar characteristic facial
deformity by virtue of their inhibiting effect on chondrocranial
growth. Certain forms of dental malocclusion also may be related to
defects of the chondrocranium.

SELECTED BIBLIOGRAPHY

BOSMA, J. F. (Ed.) (1976), *Symposium on Development of the Basicranium.*
Bethesda: U.S. Government D.H.E.W. Publication No. (NIH) 76–989.
ENLOW, D. H., and MCNAMARA, J. A. (1973), 'The Neurocranial Basis
for Facial Form and Pattern', *Angle Orthod.*, **43**, 256.
ERICSON, S., and MYRBERG, N. (1973), 'The Morphology of the Spheno-
occipital Synchondrosis at the Age of Eight Evaluated by Tomography',
Acta morph. neerl.-scand., **11**, 197.
INGERVALL, B., and THILANDER, B. (1972), 'The Human Spheno-occipital
Synchondrosis', *Acta odont. scand.*, **30**, 349.
KNOTT, VIRGINIA B. (1969), 'Ontogenetic Change of Four Cranial Base
Segments in Girls', *Growth*, **33**, 123.
— — (1971), 'Change in Cranial Base Measures of Human Males and
Females from Age 6 Years to Early Adulthood', *Ibid.*, **35**, 145.
KVINNSLAND, S. (1971), 'The Sagittal Growth of the Foetal Cranial Base',
Acta odont. scand., **29**, 699.
— — (1973), 'Changes in the Foramen Magnum Axis during Human
Foetal Life', *Ibid.*, **31**, 175.
LANG, J. (1977), 'Structure and Postnatal Organization of heretofore
Uninvestigated and Infrequent Ossifications of the Sella Turcica Region.
Acta anat., **99**, 121.
LATHAM, R. A. (1972), 'The Sella Point and Postnatal Growth of the
Human Cranial Base', *Am. J. Orthod.*, **61**, 156.
LEWIS, A. B., and ROCHE, A. F. (1974), 'Cranial Base Elongation in
Boys during Pubescence', *Angle Orthod.*, **44**, 83.
MELSEN, B. (1972), 'Time and Mode of Closure of the Spheno-occipital
Synchondrosis Determined on Human Autopsy Material', *Acta anat.*,
83, 112.
— — (1974), 'The Cranial Base. The Postnatal Development of the
Cranial Base studied Histologically on Human Autopsy Material',
Acta odont. scand., Suppl. 62, 1–126.
— — (1977), 'Histological Analysis of the Postnatal Development of the
Nasal Septum', *Angle Orthod.*, **47**, 83.

THILANDER, B., and INGERVALL, B. (1973), 'The Human Spheno-occipital Synchondrosis', *Acta odont. scand.*, **31**, 323.

TILLMAN, B., and LORENZ, R. (1978), 'The Development of the Occipital Condyle', *Anat. Embryol.*, **153**, 269.

TOERIEN, M. J., and ROSSOUW, R. J. (1977), 'Experimental Studies on the Origin of the Parts of the Nasal Capsule', *S. Afr. J. Sci.*, **73**, 371.

VAN DER LINDEN, F. P. G. M., and ENLOW, D. H. (1971), 'A Study of the Anterior Cranial Base', *Angle Orthod.*, **41**, 119.

WILSON, P. M. (1973), 'Preliminary Report on the Possible Existence of Pre-otic Sclerotomes', *S. Afr. J. Sci.*, **69**, 250.

CHAPTER 9

THE FACIAL SKELETON

THE face may be conveniently, if somewhat arbitrarily, divided into thirds—the upper, middle, and lower, their boundaries being approximately the horizontal planes passing through the pupils of the eyes and the rima oris. The three parts correspond generally to the embryonic frontonasal, maxillary, and mandibular processes respectively (p. 31). The upper third of the face is predominantly of neurocranial composition, with the frontal bone of the calvaria primarily responsible for the forehead. The middle third of the face is skeletally the most complex, being composed in part of the cranial base, and incorporating both the nasal extension of the upper third and part of the masticatory apparatus, including the maxillary dentition. The lower third of the face completes the masticatory apparatus, being composed skeletally of the mandible and its dentition.

The upper third of the face initially grows the most rapidly, in keeping with its neurocranial association and the precocious development

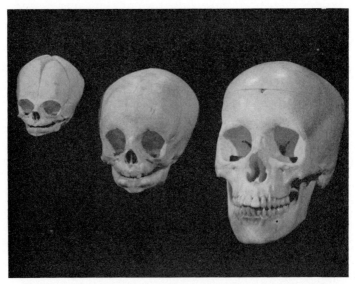

Fig. 70. Neonatal (*left*), one-year (*centre*), and adult (*right*) skulls, illustrating the relative growth of the face and neurocranium. Note the enormous expansion of the face in the adult relative to the neonate. Note the mid-mandibular and frontal sutures in the neonate.

of the frontal lobes of the brain. The upper third also achieves its ultimate growth potential at an early age, practically ceasing to grow significantly after the twelfth year of age. In contrast, the middle and lower thirds grow more slowly over a prolonged period, not ceasing growth until late adolescence (*Fig. 70*). Completion of the masticatory apparatus by the eruption of the third molars (18–25 years of age) marks the cessation of growth of the lower two-thirds of the face (*Fig. 71*).

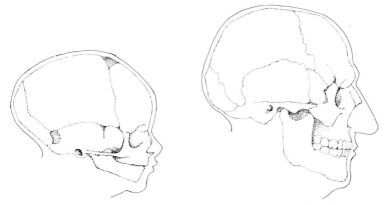

Fig. 71. Lateral aspect of the skulls of a neonate and adult illustrating the relative growth of the face and neurocranium.

The facial bones develop intramembranously from ossification centres in the neural crest mesenchyme of the embryonic facial processes (*Fig. 72* and *Frontispiece*). An interaction between the ectomesenchyme of the facial 'processes' and the overlying epithelium is believed to be a prerequisite to the differentiation of the facial bones.

The ossification centres for the upper third of the face are those of the *frontal bone*, which contributes also to the anterior part of the neurocranium. Since the frontal bone is also a component of the calvaria, details of its ossification have been described in Chapter 7 (*see* p. 80).

In the frontonasal process, intramembranous single ossification centres appear in the third month for each of the *nasal* and *lacrimal* bones in the membrane covering the cartilaginous nasal capsule. The embryonic facial maxillary processes develop numerous intramembranous ossification centres. The first ossification centres to appear early in the 8th week i.u. are those for the *medial pterygoid plates* of the *sphenoid bone* and for the *vomer*. The ossification

103

centre for the medial pterygoid plate first appears in a nodule of secondary cartilage that forms the *pterygoid hamulus*, but subsequent ossification of the pterygoid plate is intramembranous. Further intramembranous ossification centres develop for the *greater wing of the sphenoid* (in addition to its endochondral alisphenoidal centre), and for the *lateral pterygoid plate*. Bony fusion of the medial and lateral pterygoid plates takes place in the 5th month i.u. Other details of sphenoid bone development were described in Chapter 8 (*see* p. 94). Single ossification centres appear for each of the *palatine bones*, and two bilaterally for the vomer in the maxillary mesenchyme surrounding the cartilaginous nasal septum in the 8th week i.u. Further details of vomer development were described in Chapter 8 (*see* p. 89).

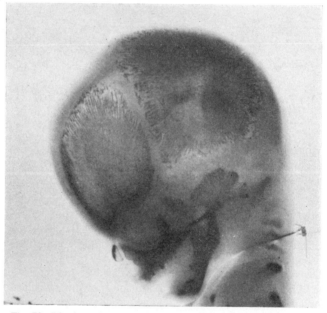

Fig. 72. The lateral aspect of the skull of a 15-week fetus stained with alizarin red and cleared to show the extent of ossification of the bones.

A primary intramembranous ossification centre appears for each *maxilla* early in the 8th week at the termination of the infraorbital nerve just above the canine tooth dental lamina. Secondary cartilages appear at the end of the 8th week in the regions of the zygomatic and alveolar processes that rapidly ossify and fuse with the primary

104

intramembranous centre. Two further intramembranous 'pre-maxillary'* centres appear anteriorly on each side in the 8th week and rapidly fuse with the primary maxillary centre.

Single ossification centres appear for each of the *zygomatic bones* and the *squamous portions of the temporal bones* in the 8th week i.u. In the lower third of the face, the mandibular processes develop bilaterally single intramembranous centres for the *mandible* and four minute centres for the *tympanic ring* of the temporal bone.

The attachment of the facial skeleton antero-inferiorly to the calvarial base determines the chondrocranial influence on facial growth. The sites of attachment are clearly defined by the pterygo-maxillary fissure and pterygopalatine fossa between the sphenoid bone of the calvarial base and the maxillary and palatine bones of the posterior aspect of the face. The zygomatic bone of the face is attached to the calvarial skeleton at the temporozygomatic and frontozygomatic sutures. The maxillary and nasal bones of the anterior aspect of the face are attached to the calvaria at the fronto-maxillary and frontonasal sutures. The interposition of three sets of space-occupying sense organs between the neural and facial skeletons complicates the attachments of these two skull compon-ents to each other, and influences the growth of the facial skeleton in particular. The eye, the nasal cavity, and its septum, and the external ear situated along the approximate boundaries of the upper and middle thirds of the face, act to a greater or lesser extent as functional matrices in determining some aspects of the growth pattern of the face. The tongue, teeth, and oromasticatory musculature are similarly interposed between the middle and lower thirds of the face, and their functioning is also influential in facial skeletal growth.

Growth of the eyes provides an expanding force separating the neural and facial skeletons, particularly at the frontomaxillary and frontozygomatic sutures, thereby contributing to skull height. The eyes appear to migrate medially from their initially lateral situation in the primitive face, due to the enormous expansion of the frontal and temporal lobes of the brain in early cranial development. The forward-directed eyes of man (and higher primates) confer a capability for stereoscopic vision and depth perception.

The eyeballs initially grow rapidly, following the neural pattern of growth and contributing to rapid widening of the fetal face. The orbits complete half their postnatal growth during the first two

---

*The existence of separate premaxillary bones in the human fetus is disputed, and the alizarin-staining loci appearing at this site are believed to be merely extensions of the maxillary primary ossification centres. The separating structure between the 'premaxilla' and maxilla is considered not to be a true suture, but a fissure. The human upper jaw accordingly develops as a single bone on each side from its inception. *See also* footnote p. 116.

years after birth, and consequently appear disproportionately large in the face of the child. The brain and the eyeball growing contemporaneously in a similarly rapid pattern 'compete' for space, and the final form of the orbital wall intervening between the two reflects mutual adjustment between these competing functional matrices. The orbital cavities attain their adult dimensions at about seven years of age.

The nasal cavity, and in particular the nasal septum, have considerable influence in determining facial form. In the fetus, a septo-maxillary ligament arising from the sides and anteroinferior border of the nasal septum, and inserting into the anterior nasal spine, transmits septal growth 'pull' upon the maxilla. Facial growth is directed downwards and forwards by the septal cartilage that between the 10th and 40th weeks i.u. grows sevenfold in vertical length. The nasal cavity at birth lies almost entirely between the orbits. Nasal septal cartilage growth continues postnatally at a decreasing rate during the first 6 years of life, thereby lowering the nasal cavity floor below the orbits.

The 'thrust' and 'pull' created by nasal septal growth separate to varying degrees the frontomaxillary, frontonasal, frontozygomatic, and zygomaticomaxillary sutures. Dramatic demonstration of the growth potential of the nasal septal cartilage is provided in cases of bilateral cleft lip and palate, where the tip of the nose, columella, philtrum, prolabium and primary palate form a 'proboscis' which, freed from its lateral attachments to the maxillae, protrudes conspicuously on the face as a result of vomerine and nasal septal growth (*Fig. 42*, p. 47). This growth thrust is normally dissipated into adjacent facial structures. It is of interest to note that the nasal septum does not deflect from the midline until adolescence, when facial growth normally ceases, and the nasal septum then commonly becomes deflected. The expansion of the eyeballs, the brain, and the spheno-occipital synchondrosal cartilage also act variably in separating the facial sutures. Furthermore, the situation of these sutures later subjects them to forces exerted by the masticatory muscles, in having to buttress against masticatory pressures transmitted through the adjacent bones.

Growth of the maxilla is dependent upon a number of functional matrices acting upon different areas of the bone that theoretically allows its subdivision into 'skeletal units' (*Fig. 73*). The 'basal body' develops beneath the infraorbital nerve, later surrounding it to form the infraorbital canal. The 'orbital unit' responds to the growth of the eyeball. The 'nasal unit' is dependent upon the septal cartilage for its growth, while the teeth provide the functional matrix for the 'alveolar unit'. The 'pneumatic unit' reflects maxillary sinus expansion, which is more a responder than determiner of

106

this skeletal unit. Development of the maxillary sinus is further described in Chapter 11 (*see* p. 124).

The complexity of all these functional forces acting on the facial bones produces different effects on different sutures (*Fig. 74*). Thus, the temporozygomatic suture in the zygomatic arch has been shown to have a predominantly anteroposterior horizontal direction of growth, largely due to the longitudinal growth of the brain and the spheno-occipital synchondrosal cartilage. The anteroposterior growth at the nasomaxillary sutures, creating the elevated bridge of

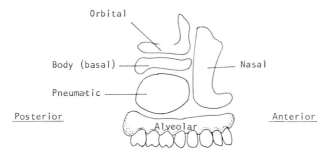

Fig. 73. Schema of 'skeletal units' of the maxilla.

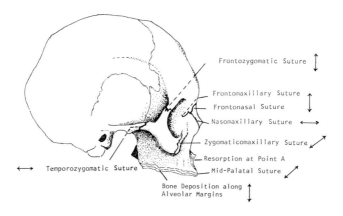

Fig. 74. Directions of growth and resorption of the facial bones at various sites. The overall effect of the combination of these growth sites is a downward and forward displacement of the face *vis-à-vis* the cranial base.

the nose, would result from anteroposterior nasal septal expansion. The frontomaxillary, frontozygomatic, frontonasal, ethmoidomaxillary and fronto-ethmoidal sutures are the sites of bone growth in a largely vertical direction, as a result of eyeball and nasal septal expansion. Should the nasal septum be defective in its growth, the height of the middle third of the face is not as seriously affected as is its anteroposterior dimension, resulting in a concave appearance to the face. Lateral expansion of the zygomaticomaxillary sutures by the eyes, and growth at the intermaxillary suture, contribute to the widening of the face. The width of the neonate face is relatively less in proportion to the neurocranium than it is in the adult. The face of the newborn is twice as broad in comparison to its height than in the adult, and adjusts to adult proportions during the childhood years.

The overall effect of these diverse directions of growth is osseous accretion predominantly on the posterior and superior surfaces of the facial bones. Encapsulated fatty tissue, interposed between the posterosuperior surfaces of the maxilla and the cranial base (sphenoid bone), provides a compression-resisting structure. Bone deposition on the posterosuperior maxillary surface and in the maxillary alveolar tuberosity region results in a displacement of the maxilla away from this retromaxillary fat pad. With fat pads and the chondrocranium acting as a base against which facial bone growth takes place, the result is that the middle (and as will be seen later, the lower) third of the face moves in a marked downward and slightly forward direction *vis-à-vis* the cranial base. Growth at these suture sites occurs most markedly up to the fourth year of life postnatally. Thereafter, these sutures function mainly as sites of fibrous union of the skull bones, allowing for adjustments brought about by surface apposition and remodelling

Remodelling takes place on all the bone surfaces to adjust the bones to their altered positions as a result of displacement. Of particular interest is the deposition of bone along the alveolar margins of the maxillae (and mandible) within which incipient alveolar processes the tooth germs are developing. When tooth germs are congenitally absent, the alveolar processes fail to develop. The growth of the alveolar processes adds considerably to the vertical height of the face and to the depth of the palate, and allows concomitant expansion of the maxillary sinuses. Bone deposition on the posterior surface of the maxillary tuberosity produces corresponding anterior displacement of the whole maxilla. The eruption of the teeth through the alveolar process accentuates the vertical and posterior growth of the maxillae. The dental alveolar arch growth pattern differs from that of the facial skeleton, however, by being related to the sequence of tooth eruption. Resorption along the anterior surface of the bodies of the maxillae creates the supra-alveolar concavity, known as Point A in orthodontic parlance, thus emphasizing the projection of the anterior nasal spine of the maxilla.

The empty space of the nasal cavity may also influence facial growth and form. Inadequate use of the nasal cavity by mouth breathing has been associated with the narrow pinched face and highly vaulted palatal arch of the 'adenoidal facies', so called because of the once believed association with hypertrophied pharyngeal tonsils or 'adenoids'. The cause and effect relationship of this particular (?inherited) facial form with mouth breathing, if any, has not been adequately substantiated.

The role of the ear, as a space-occupying sense organ, is somewhat of an ambiguous one in influencing facial form, and would appear to be minimal. The otic capsule that houses the vestibulocochlear apparatus completes its ossification from four centres to form the petrous temporal bone at the time that the internal ear reaches its adult size, in the latter part of the fifth and early in the sixth month of fetal life. The inner ear is the only organ that reaches full adult size by this age. This early completion of the inner ear mini-mizes its influence on subsequent growth of the cranial skeleton. However, the situation of the inner and middle ears in the floor of the cranial cavity necessarily results in the vestibulocochlear organ encroaching on the brain space between the middle and posterior endocranial fossae. Together with the deposition of osseous tissue on the endocranial surface of the petrous temporal bone, the infringement of the inner and middle ears on the brain space may cause compensatory increases of the cranial cavity in other directions.

Abnormal Development

Malformations of the face may arise from aberrations of morpho-genesis at many levels of development, and may be genetically or environmentally determined. The basis of many congenital abnor-malities begins with maldevelopment of neural crest tissue that gives rise to much of the skeletal and connective tissue primordia of the face. Neural crest cells may be deficient in number, or may not migrate fully to their destination, or fail in their inductive capacity. A failure of ectoderm or endoderm matrix to respond to neural crest induction may also be responsible for facial defects.

Absent or insufficient neural crest ectomesenchyme in the fronto-nasal process may be responsible for cleft lips. Deficiencies of maxillary process and branchial arch ectomesenchyme (possibly because of the long path of neural crest migration) may result in absent facial bones. The clinical syndrome of mandibulofacial dysostosis (Treacher-Collins syndrome) that exhibits a sunken appearance of the cheeks is due to severe hypoplasia or absence of the zygomatic bones. Deficient facial bone development in anhidrotic ectodermal dysplasia that displays a 'dished' face may reflect defective ectodermal-neural crest induction mechanisms. Down's syndrome (trisomy 21) features less proclined and shortened or even absent nasal bones, accounting for the 'saddle nose' so characteristic of this affliction. The maxilla in Down's syndrome is furthermore much smaller than normal, being reduced most in width. Deficient maxillary development may be associated with clefts of the upper lip and palate (*Fig. 75*).

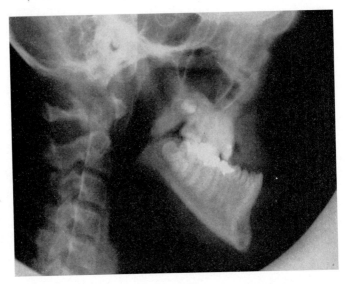

Fig. 75. Radiograph of deficient maxillary development in a 16-year-old boy who also manifested a unilateral right side cleft lip and palate. The mandible is overgrown, exaggerating the discrepancy between the lower and middle thirds of the face.

Inadequate diencephalic brain development at a very early stage results in the primordial optic vesicles developing close to each other, and fusing to form a single median eye (*cyclops*) (*see Fig. 40*, p. 45). This gross developmental defect does not allow for survival. In normal development, the distance separating the eyes greatly influences the 'character' of the face. A narrow interocular distance confers a sharp 'foxy' appearance to the face. The condition of ocular *hypertelorism* is characterized by an abnormally great interorbital distance separating the eyes, tending to confer a 'wide-eyed' appearance. This mild developmental defect is due to an embryological morphokinetic arrest that leaves the orbits in a fetal position. The nasal bones and the cribriform plate of the ethmoid remain especially widened, and the sphenoid bone is enlarged.

The ectomesenchymal and mesodermal deficiencies producing these abnormalities are mainly caused by chromosomal anomalies and mutant genes, but environmental factors are possibly involved in some cases. Facial clefts, including those afflicting the lips and palate, are components of over 100 syndromes. Many of these syndromes exhibit single gene inheritance.

Unilateral defective facial development, known as *hemifacial microsomia* produces an asymmetrical face. The underdeveloped structures are the ear, including the ear ossicles (*microtia*), the zygomatic bone and mandible of one side of the face. The parotid gland, tongue and facial muscles are also unilaterally defective. The cause of this condition has been traced to a destructive haematoma emanating from the primitive stapedial artery at about the 32nd day of development.

Congenital excrescences of abnormal facial growth may occur as midline frontal or nasal masses. They encompass *encephalocoeles*, *gliomas* and *dermoid cysts*. Congenital invaginations of the face constitute *dermal sinuses* and *fistulae*. Intracranial communication of these facial defects often exists due to cranial bone deficiencies. Herniation of the intracranial contents through the frontonasal, fronto-ethmoidal or frontosphenoidal complexes occurs due to failure of closure of the foramen caecum of the ethmoid-frontal bone junction (*see* p. 80).

Other defects of facial development have been dealt with on p. 46.

SELECTED BIBLIOGRAPHY

AITA, J. A. (1969), *Congenital Facial Anomalies with Neurological Defects*. Springfield, Ill.: Thomas.

BERGLAND, O., and BORCHGREVINK, H. (1974), 'The Role of the Nasal Septum in Midfacial Growth in Man Elucidated by the Maxillary Development in Certain Types of Facial Clefts', *Scand. J. Plast. Reconstr. Surg.*, **8**, 42.

BJÖRK, A., and SKIELLER, V. (1974), 'Growth in Width of the Maxilla Studied by the Implant Method', *Ibid.*, **8**, 26.

BRODIE, A. G. (1971), 'Emerging Concepts of Facial Growth', *Angle Orthod.*, **41**, 103.

CANNON, J. (1970), 'Craniofacial Height and Depth Increments in Normal Children', *Ibid.*, **40**, 202.

ENLOW, D. H. (1968), *The Human Face. An Account of the Postnatal Growth and Development of the Craniofacial Skeleton*. New York: Harper & Row.

111

ENLOW, D. H., and MOYERS, R. E. (1971), 'Growth and Architecture of the Face', *J. Am. dent. Ass.*, **82**, 763.

GARDNER, D. G., and LIM, H. (1971), 'The Oral Manifestations of Cyclopia', *Oral Surg.*, **32**, 910.

GLASS, D. F. (1966), 'Unilateral Craniofacial Deformities', *Dent. Practnr dent. Rec.*, **16**, 179.

— — (1970), 'The Recognition of Bilateral Craniofacial Deformities', *Ibid.*, **21**, 137.

GOODMAN, R. M., and GORLIN, R. J. (1977), *The Face in Genetic Disorders*, 2nd ed., St. Louis: Mosby.

GORLIN, R. J., PINDBORG, J. J., and COHEN, M. M. (1975), *Syndromes of the Head and Neck*, 2nd ed., New York: McGraw-Hill.

HARVEY-KEMBLE, J. V. (1973), 'The Importance of the Nasal Septum in Facial Development'. *J. Laryng. Otol.*, **87**, 379.

HIXON, E. H. (1970), 'Development of the Facial Complex'. Chapter in: *Proceedings of the Workshop on Speech and the Dentofacial Complex: The State of the Art. Report No. 5.* Washington: American Speech and Hearing Association, pp. 33–48.

JOHNSTON, M. C., and PRATT, R. M. (1975), 'The Neural Crest in Normal and Abnormal Craniofacial Development'. Chap. 71 in *Extracellular Matrix Influences of Gene Expression.* (Ed. SLAVKIN, H. C., and GREULICH, R. C.). New York: Academic Press.

KRAUS, B. S., and DECKER, J. D. (1960), 'The Prenatal Inter-relationships of the Maxilla and Premaxilla in the Facial Development of Man', *Acta anat.*, **40**, 278.

KVINNSLAND, S. (1969), 'Observations on the Early Ossification of the Upper Jaw', *Acta odont. scand.*, **27**, 649.

— — (1971), 'The Sagittal Growth of the Upper Face during Foetal Life', *Ibid.*, **29**, 717.

LATHAM, R. A. (1970), 'Maxillary Development and Growth. The Septo-premaxillary Ligament', *J. Anat.*, **107**, 471.

LINDNER-ARONSON, S., and BACKSTROM, A. (1960), 'A Comparison between Mouth and Nose Breathers with Respect to Occlusion and Facial Dimensions', *Odont. Rev.*, **11**, 343.

MAZZOLA, R. F. (1976), 'Congenital Malformations in the Frontonasal Area: Their Pathogenesis and Classification', *Clin. in Plast. Surg.*, **3**, 573.

MCNAMARA, J. A. (Ed.) (1976), *Factors Affecting the Growth of the Midface* Monograph No. 6, Craniofacial Growth Series. Ann Arbor: University of Michigan.

MEREDITH, H. V. (1960), 'Changes in Form of the Head and Face during Childhood', *Growth*, **24**, 215.

— — and KNOTT, V. B. (1973), *Childhood Changes of Head, Face and Dentition.* Iowa City: Iowa Orthodontic Society.

MICHEJDA, M. (1972), 'The Role of Basicranial Synchondroses in Flexure Processes and Ontogenetic Development of the Skull Base', *Am. J. Phys. Anthropol.*, **37**, 143.

MILLARD, D. R. Jr. (1976), *Cleft Craft.* Boston: Little, Brown and Co.

MOORE, W. J., and LAVELLE, C. L. B. (1974), *Growth of the Facial Skeleton in the Hominoidea.* New York: Academic Press.

OBWEGESER, H. L., WEBER, G., FREIHOFER, H. P., and SAILER, H. F. (1978), 'Facial Duplication—the Unique Case of Antonio', *J. Maxillofac. Surg.*, **6,** 179.

POSWILLO, D. (1975), 'The Pathogenesis of the Treacher Collins Syndrome (Mandibulofacial Dysostosis)', *Br. J. oral Surg.*, **13,** 1.

PRUZANSKY, S. (1961), (Ed.) *Congenital Anomalies of the Face and Associated Structures.* Springfield, Ill.: Thomas.

— — (1971), 'The Growth of the Premaxillary-Vomerine Complex in Complete Bilateral Cleft Lip and Palate', *Tandlaegebladet,* **75,** 1157.

SARNAT, B. G. (1963), 'Post-natal Growth of the Upper Face: Some Experimental Considerations', *Angle Orthod.*, **33,** 139.

SCOTT, J. H. (1953), 'The Cartilage of the Nasal Septum. A Contribution to the Study of Facial Growth', *Br. dent. J.*, **95,** 37.

TESSIER, P. (1976), 'Anatomical Classification of Facial, Craniofacial and Laterofacial Clefts', *J. Maxillofac. Surg.*, **4,** 69.

TULLEY, W. J. (1964), 'Malformation of the Jaws and Teeth in Relation to Upper Respiratory Symptoms and Certain Speech Disorders', *Guy's Hosp. Rep.*, **113** (3,4), 261.

WALKER. D. G. (1961), *Malformations of the Face.* Edinburgh: Livingstone.

CHAPTER 10

THE PALATE

THE human palate in its embryological development passes through stages representing divisions of the oronasal chamber found in primitive crossopterygian fish, reptiles and early mammals. The history of the separation of the respiratory and masticatory functions of the stomodeal chamber is thereby briefly recapitulated.

The three elements that make up the secondary definitive palate—the two lateral maxillary palatal shelves and the primary palate of the frontonasal process—are initially widely separated due to the vertical orientation of the lateral shelves on either side of the tongue (*see Figs. 30, 33*, pp. 39, 41). Late in the 7th week i.u. (between the 47th and 54th days) a remarkable transformation in position of the lateral shelves takes place, when they alter from vertical to horizontal, as a prelude to their fusion and partitioning the oronasal chamber (*Fig. 76*).

The transition from the vertical to the horizontal position takes place within hours.* Several mechanisms have been proposed for the rapid elevation of the palatal shelves. This movement has been variously ascribed to biochemical transformations in the physical consistency of the connective tissue matrix of the palatal shelves; to variations in vasculature and blood flow to these structures; to rapid differential mitotic growth; to an 'intrinsic shelf force'; and to muscular movements. The withdrawal of the embryo's face from against the heart prominence by uprighting of the head facilitates jaw opening. Mouth-opening reflexes have been implicated in the withdrawal of the tongue from between the vertical shelves, and pressure differences between the nasal and oral regions due to tongue muscle contraction may account for palatal shelf elevation.

The epithelium overlying the edges of the palatal shelves is especially thickened, and their fusion upon mutual contact is crucial to intact palatal development. Fusion also occurs between the dorsal surfaces of the fusing palatal processes and the lower edge of the midline nasal septum. The mechanisms of adhesive contact, fusion and subsequent degeneration of the epithelium are presently not clearly understood. A combination of degenerating surface cells and an epithelial surface coat accumulation of polyanionic substances such as glycoprotein may facilitate epithelial adherence

---

*There is a considerable sex difference in the timing of human palatal closure. Shelf elevation and fusion begins a few days earlier in male than in female embryos, possibly accounting for sex differences in the incidence of cleft palates.

between contacting palatal processes. It appears that programmed cell death of the fused epithelium is an essential prerequisite for mesenchymal coalescence of the shelves to occur. The epithelium at the leading edges of the palatal shelves may contribute to failure of fusion by not breaking down after shelf approximation, leading to 'epithelial pearl' formation, or by not maintaining an 'adhesiveness' beyond a critical time should palatal shelf elevation be delayed.

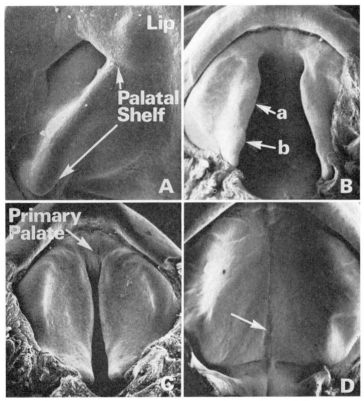

Fig. 76. A, View of left half of stomodeum of 6-week human embryo showing early vertical palatal shelf and lip forming from the maxillary process. Note the blunt, rounded posterior end. S.E.M. ×30. B, View of the palatal shelves of a 7-week human embryo showing the anterior end of the right shelf (*a*) becoming horizontal, while the posterior end of the shelf (*b*) remains vertical. S.E.M. ×11. C, View of the palatal shelves of an 8-week human embryo showing the completely horizontal shelves approaching each other in the midline. S.E.M. ×11. D, The nearly fused lateral palatal shelves of a 9-week human embryo showing fusion with the primary palate anteriorly. The soft palate region (arrow) is still unfused. S.E.M. ×8. (*Scanning electron photomicrographs by courtesy of Drs R. E. Waterman and S. M. Meller and the Wistar Institute Press.*)

115

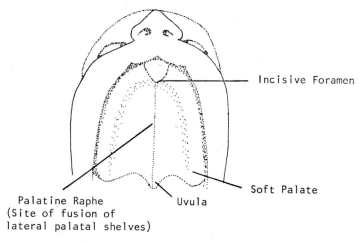

Fig. 77. Lines of fusion of the embryological primordia of the palate.

The fusion of the three palatal processes initially produces a flat, unarched roof to the mouth. The fusing lateral palatal shelves overlap the anterior primary palate as indicated later by the sloping pathways of the junctional incisive neurovascular canals that carry the previously formed incisive nerves and blood-vessels. The site of junction of the three palatal components is marked by the incisive papilla overlying the incisive canal. The line of fusion of the lateral palatal shelves is traced in the adult by the midpalatal suture,* and on the surface by the midline raphe of the hard palate (*Figs. 77, 78*). This fusion 'seam' is minimized in the soft palate by extra-territorial mesenchymal invasion.

Ossification of the palate proceeds during the 8th week i.u. from the spread of bone into the mesenchyme of the fused lateral palatal shelves and from trabeculae appearing in the primary palate as 'premaxillary centres',† all derived from the single primary ossification centres of the maxillae. Posteriorly, the hard palate is ossified

---

*Inclusive of the palatal portion of the intermaxillary suture and the median palatine suture between the two palatine bones.

†The human premaxilla is believed not to exist as a separate entity, in contra-distinction to its existence in most mammalian and primate upper jaws. The bone formed by the 4 premaxillary 'ossification centres' (2 on each side) is over-grown superficially by the maxillary bone, eliminating evidence of a premaxilla from the facial aspect after the 3rd month i.u. However, a fissure occasionally may be seen on the palatal aspect, running between the lateral incisor and canine teeth to the incisive fossa, producing a so-called *os incisivum*. *See also* footnote, p. 105.

from the trabeculae spreading from the single primary ossification centres of each of the palatine bones.

Midpalatal sutural structure is first evident at 10½ weeks when an upper layer of fibre bundles develops across the midline. The palatine bone elements of the palate remain separated from the maxillary elements by the palatomaxillary sutures into adulthood.

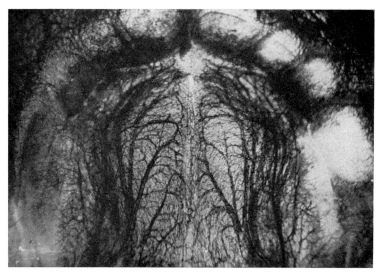

Fig. 78. Photomicrograph of the palate of a human 6-month fetus. Bone removed by microdissection and the arteries and capillaries injected with india ink. Note the midline raphe and the arterial anastomotic arcades, with only capillaries crossing over the midline. The tooth buds in the dental arch are outlined by the surrounding vascular networks. (*By courtesy of Dr William P. Maher.*)

In the most posterior part of the palate ossification does not occur, giving rise to the region of the soft palate. Branchiomeric mesenchymal tissue of the first and fourth branchial arches migrates into this faucial region, supplying the musculature of the soft palate and the fauces. The tensor veli palatini is derived from the first arch, and the levator veli palatini, uvular and faucial pillar muscles from the fourth arch, accounting for the innervation by the trigeminal nerve of the tensor veli palatini muscle, and by the vagus nerve for all the other muscles (*Fig. 79*).

Growth of the hard palate takes place in length, breadth, and height, converting it into an arched roof for the mouth (*Fig. 80*). The fetal palate initially increases in length more rapidly than in width between 7 and 18 weeks i.u. Subsequently, growth in width

117

overtakes that in length. In early prenatal life the palate is relatively long, but from the 4th month i.u. onwards, it becomes wider as a result of midpalatal sutural growth and appositional growth along the lateral alveolar margins. At birth, the length and breadth of the hard palate are almost equal. The later postnatal increase of palatal length is due to appositional growth in the maxillary tuberosity region, and, to some extent, at the transverse palatine suture.

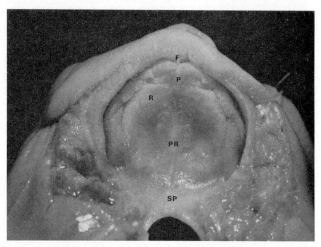

Fig. 79. Palate and upper lip of a 22-week-old fetus. Note the midline frenum (F), the papilla (P) overlying the incisive foramen, and the grooved alveolar arch divided into segments containing the developing tooth buds. The palatine raphe (PR) marks the site of patatal shelf fusion. The rugae (R) become more prominent towards birth. The soft palate (SP) is extensive.

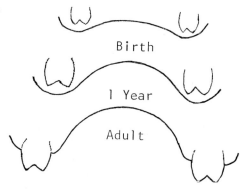

Fig. 80. Cross-sectional views of the palate at different ages. Note the increasing depth of the palatal arch concomitant with tooth eruption.

118

Growth at the midpalatal suture ceases between one and two years of age although no synostosis occurs to signify cessation of its growth.* Growth in width of the midpalatal suture is larger in its posterior than in its anterior part, so that the posterior part of the nasal cavity widens more than its anterior part. Obliteration of the midpalatal suture may start in adolescence, but complete fusion is rarely found before 30 years of age. Great variability exists in the timing and degree of fusion of this suture.

Appositional lateral growth occurs in the palate up until seven years of age, at which age the palate achieves its ultimate anterior width. Appositional growth continues posteriorly after lateral growth has ceased, accounting for a lengthening of the palate over its width during late childhood. During infancy and childhood, bone apposition also occurs on the entire inferior surface of the palate, accompanied by concomitant resorption from its superior (nasal) surface. The result of this bone remodelling is descent of the palate, and enlargement of the nasal cavity. Increase of nasal capacity must keep pace with general body growth that determines increasing respiratory requirements. A fundamental drive in facial growth is provision of an adequate nasal capacity, that if not met, is diverted to the mouth for maintenance of respiration.

The appositional growth of the alveolar processes contributes to a deepening, as well as a widening, of the vault of the bony palate, at the same time adding to the height and breadth of the maxillae. The lateral alveolar processes help to form an anteroposterior palatal furrow, which, together with a concave floor produced by a tongue curled from side to side, results in a palatal tunnel ideally suited to receive a nipple. A variable number of transverse *palatal rugae* develop in the mucosa covering the hard palate. The rugae are most prominent in the infant, and are useful for holding the nipple while it is being milked by the tongue. The anterior palatal furrow is well marked during the first year of life, concomitant with the active suckling period, and normally flattens out into the palatal arch after three to four years of age when suckling has been discontinued. Persistence of thumb or finger-sucking habits may retain the accentuated palatal furrow into childhood.

Anomalies of Palatal Development

Successful fusion of the three embryonic components of the palate involves a complicated synchronization of shelf movements with tongue growth and withdrawal, and with mandibular and head

---

*The retention of a syndesmosis in the midpalatal suture into adulthood, even after growth has normally ceased at this site, allows for orthodontic palatal expansion therapy to be successfully applied. Forceful separation of the suture by an orthodontic appliance reinstitutes compensatory bone growth at this site.

growth. Mis-timing of any of these critical events, either by environmental agents or genetic predisposition, will result in failure of fusion, leading to clefts of the palate of varying degrees of severity.

The entrapment of epithelial 'rests' or 'pearls' in the line of fusion of the palatal shelves, particularly the midline raphe of the hard palate, may later give rise to median palatal 'rest' cysts. A frequent superficial expression of these epithelial entrapments are epithelial cysts or nodules known as *Epstein's pearls* that occur along the median raphe of the hard palate and at the junction of the hard and soft palates. Small *mucosal gland retention cysts* (*Bohn's nodules*) may occur on the buccal and lingual aspects of the alveolar ridges, while *dental lamina cysts* may develop on the crests of the alveolar ridges from epithelial remnants of the dental lamina. All these superficial cysts of the palate in the newborn usually disappear by the third postnatal month. An anterior midline maxillary cyst developing in the region of the primary palate cannot be of fissural origin, but is a *nasopalatine duct cyst* encroaching anteriorly into the palate. Cysts are rare in the soft palate because of the mesenchymal merging of the shelves in this region.

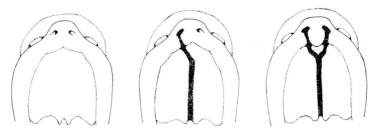

Fig. 81. Schema of degrees of clefting of the palate. *Left:* bifid uvula. *Centre:* unilateral cleft palate and lip. *Right:* bilateral cleft palate and lip.

Delay in the elevation of the palatal shelves from the vertical to the horizontal (p. 114), while the head is continually growing, will result in the shelves being too far apart to meet, and fuse, in the midline when eventually they do become horizontal leading to clefting of the palate.

The least severe form of cleft palate is the bifid uvula, of relatively frequent occurrence. Increasingly severe clefts always incur posterior involvement, the cleft advancing anteriorly in contradistinction to the direction of normal fusion (*Fig. 81*). The lines of fusion of the lateral palatal shelves with the primary palate dictate the diversion from the midline of a severe palatal cleft anteriorly to either the right or the left, or to both, in rare instances. If the cleft involves the alveolar arch, it usually passes between the lateral incisor and canine teeth. Such severe cleft palates may or may not be associated with unilateral or bilateral cleft upper lips, in that the two conditions are independently determined. The vertical nasal septum may fuse with either the left or the right palatal shelf, or with neither, in cases of severe cleft palate (*Figs. 82, 83*).

Clefts of the soft palate alone incur varying degrees of speech difficulty and minor swallowing problems because of the inability to close off completely the oropharynx from the nasopharynx during

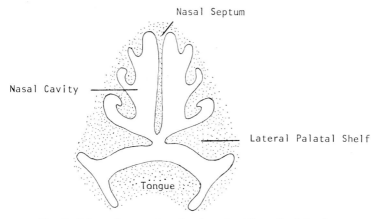

Fig. 82. Schematic coronal section through a bilaterally cleft palate, with an oral opening into both nasal cavities.

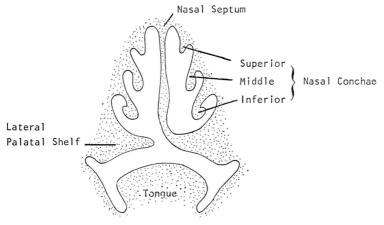

Fig. 83. Schematic coronal section through a unilateral cleft palate with an oral opening into one nasal cavity only.

121

these pharyngeal functions. Clefts of the hard palate, which almost invariably includes soft palate clefts, produce feeding problems of varying severity, particularly in the infant, whose vacuum-producing suckling processes demand an intact hard palate. Spillage of food into the nasal fossa(e) is symptomatic of feeding difficulties. Early reparative surgery and/or obturator fitting is accordingly indicated for afflicted infants' nutritional well-being, and later, for correct speech enunciation. Cleft palate constitutes a feature of a number of congenital defect syndromes among which are mandibulofacial dysostosis (Treacher-Collins syndrome), micrognathia (Pierre Robin syndrome), and orodigitofacial dysostosis. The palate is narrower, shorter and lower than normal in Down's syndrome (trisomy 21) although it is often described as displaying a high midline elevation, combined with a horizontal flattening laterally along the alveolar ridges, to create a 'steeple palate'. A highly arched palate is also characteristic of Marfan's syndrome, an inherited disorder manifesting skeletal and cardiovascular anomalies, in which hyperchondroplasia is a feature, but which paradoxically manifests a short nasal septal cartilage. Cleidocranial dysostosis, a congenital defect of intramembranous bones, also manifests a highly arched, and occasionally cleft, palate. Other congenital conditions displaying a high arched palate are craniofacial dysostosis (Crouzon's syndrome), acrocephalosyndactyly (Apert's syndrome), progeria, Turner's syndrome (XO sex chromosome complement), and oculodentodigital dysplasia.

A not uncommon genetically determined anomaly of the palate is a localized midpalatal overgrowth of bone of varying size known as a *torus palatinus*. When present, it reaches its greatest expression in adulthood, and while it has no direct influence on dental occlusion, a prominent torus palatinus may interfere with the seating of a removable orthodontic appliance or an upper denture.

SELECTED BIBLIOGRAPHY
ADUSS, H. (1971), 'Craniofacial Growth in Complete Unilateral Cleft Lip and Palate', *Angle Orthod.*, **41**, 202.

BURDI, A. R. and FAIST, K. (1967), 'Morphogenesis of the Palate in Normal Human Embryos with Special Emphasis on the Mechanisms Involved', *Am. J. Anat.*, **120**, 149.

BURKE, G. W., FEAGANS, W. M., ELZAY, R. P., and SCHWARTZ, L. D. (1966), 'Some Aspects of the Origin and Fate of Midpalatal Cysts in Human Fetuses', *J. dent. Res.*, **45**, 159.

DAVIS, W. M., and KRONMAN, J. H. (1969), 'Anatomical Changes Induced by Splitting of the Midpalatal Suture', *Angle Orthod.*, **39**, 126.

DICKSON, D. R., GRANT, J. C. B., SICHER, H., DUBRUL, E. L., and PALTAN, J. (1974–5), 'Status of Research in Cleft Palate Anatomy and Physiology, July 1973', *Cleft Palate J.*, **11**, 471 and **12**, 131.

EKSTRÖM, C., HENRIKSON, C. O. and JENSEN, R. (1977), 'Mineralization in the Midpalatal Suture after Orthodontic Expansion', *Am. J. Orthod.*, **71**, 449.

FREDERIKS, E. (1972), 'Vascular patterns in Normal and Cleft Primary and Secondary Palate in Human Embryos', *Br. J. Plast. Surg.*, **25**, 207.

GOSS, A. N. (1975), 'Human Palatal Development *in Vitro*', *Cleft Palate J.*, **12**, 210.

GREENE, R. M. and PRATT, R. M. (1976), 'Developmental Aspects of Secondary Palate Formation', *J. Embryol. exp. Morph.*, **36**, 225.

HUMPHREY, T. (1969), 'The Relation between Human Fetal Mouth Opening Reflexes and Closure of the Palate, *Am. J. Anat.*, **125**, 317.

JACOBSON, A. (1955), 'Embryological Evidence for the Non-existence of the Premaxilla in Man', *J. Dent. Assoc. S. Afr.*, **10**, 189.

KNOTT, V. B. (1970), 'Height and Shape of the Palate in Girls: A Longitudinal Study', *Archs oral Biol.*, **15**, 849.

LATHAM, R. A. (1971), 'The Development, Structure and Growth Pattern of the Human Midpalatal Suture', *J. Anat.*, **108**, 31.

LEBRET, L. (1962), 'Growth Changes of the Palate', *J. dent. Res.*, **41**, 1391.

LUKE, D. A. (1976), 'Development of the Secondary Palate in Man', *Acta anat.*, **94**, 596.

MELLER, S. M. and BARTON, C. H. (1978), 'Extracellular Coat in Developing Human Palatal Processes: Electron Microscopy and Ruthenium Red Binding', *Anat. Rec.*, **190**, 223.

MELSEN, B. (1975), 'Palatal Growth Studied on Human Autopsy Material', *Am. J. Orthod.*, **68**, 42.

PERSSON, M. and THILANDER, B. (1977), 'Palatal Suture Closure in Man from 15–35 years of Age', *Am. J. Orthod.*, **72**, 42.

POSWILLO, D. (1974), 'The Pathogenesis of Submucous Cleft Palate', *Scand. J. Plast. Reconstr. Surg.*, **8**, 34.

REDMAN, R. S., SHAPIRO, B. L., and GORLIN, R. J. (1965), 'Measurement of Normal and Reportedly Malformed Palatal Vaults III: Down's Syndrome (Trisomy 21 Mongolism)', *J. Paediat.*, **67**, 162.

ROSS, R. B., and JOHNSTON, M. C. (1972), *Cleft Lip and Palate*. Baltimore: Williams & Wilkins.

SCOTT, J. (1968), 'The Development, Structure, and Function of Alveolar Bone', *Dent. Practnr dent. Rec.*, **19**, 19.

SHAPIRO, B. L., GORLIN, R. J., REDMAN, R. S., and BRUHL, H. H. (1967), 'The Palate and Down's Syndrome', *New Engl. J. Med.*, **276**, 1460.

SMILEY, G. R. (1975), 'A Histological Study of the Formation and Development of the Soft Palate in Mice and Man', *Archs oral Biol.*, **20**, 297.

VIDIC, B. (1968), 'The Structure of the Palatum Osseum and its Toral Overgrowths', *Acta Anat.*, **71**, 94.

WATERMAN, R. E., and MELLER, S. M. (1974), 'Alterations in the Epithelial Surface of Human Palatal Shelves Prior to and During Fusion: A Scanning Electron Microscopic Study', *Anat. Rec.*, **180**, 111.

WOOD, P. J., and KRAUS, B. S. (1962), 'Prenatal Development of the Human Palate', *Archs oral Biol.*, **7**, 137.

WOOD, N. K., WRAGG, L. E., STUTTEVILLE, O. H., and OGLESBY, R. J. (1969), 'Osteogenesis of the Human Upper Jaw: Proof of the Non-existence of a Separate Premaxillary Centre'. *Archs oral Biol.*, **14**, 1331.

CHAPTER 11

THE PARANASAL SINUSES

THE four sets of paranasal sinuses—maxillary, sphenoidal, frontal, and ethmoidal—begin their development at the end of the third month i.u. as outpouchings of the mucous membranes of the middle, superior, and supreme nasal meatuses, and the spheno-ethmoidal recesses. The early paranasal sinuses expand into the walls and roof of the nasal fossae by growth of mucous membrane sacs into

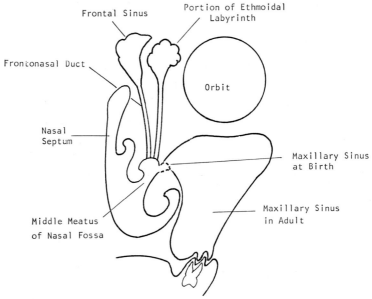

Fig. 84. Coronal sectional schema of frontal, ethmoidal and maxillary sinuses.

the maxillary, sphenoid, frontal, and ethmoid bones. The sinuses enlarge variably and greatly from their initial small outpocketings, but always retain their original communication with the nasal fossae through *ostia* (*Fig. 84*).

Pneumatization of the paranasal bones occurs at different rates, with the maxillary sinus being the earliest (at 3 months i.u.) and most precocious, and achieving a sufficiently large size at birth* to be of

---

*The maxillary sinus averages 7 mm. in length and 4 mm. in height and width at birth, and expands approximately 2 mm. vertically and 3 mm. antero-posteriorly each year.

clinical importance and radiographically identifiable. The maxillary sinus enlarges by bone resorption of the maxilla's internal walls (except medially) at a rate a little greater than overall maxillary growth. Sinus expansion causes resorption of cancellous bone except on the medial wall, where internal bone deposition is matched by opposing nasal surface resorption, thereby enlarging the nasal cavity. The rapid and continuous downwards growth of this sinus after birth brings its walls in close proximity to the roots of the maxillary cheek teeth, and its floor below its osteal opening. As each tooth erupts, the vacated bone becomes pneumatized by the expanding maxillary sinus. In adulthood, the roots of the molar teeth frequently project into the sinus lumen.

The sphenoidal sinuses commence at the 4th month i.u. by invading the posterior part of the nasal capsule into the body of the sphenoid bone. It continues growing into early adulthood, and may invade the wings, and rarely, the pterygoid plates of the sphenoid bone.

The ethmoidal air cells invade the ethmoid bone from the nasal fossa as groups of 3–15 air cells on each side from the 5th month i.u. They may be of a clinically significant size at birth. The ethmoid air cells grow variably into irregular contours (the ethmoid labyrinth) until puberty (*Fig. 85*). The most anterior of the ethmoidal cells grow upward into the frontal bone, and may form the frontal sinuses, retaining their origin from the middle meatus of the nose as the frontonasal duct. Expansion of the ethmoidal air cells may also take place into the sphenoid, lacrimal or even maxillary bones where they are designated extramural sphenoidal, lacrimal or maxillary sinuses.

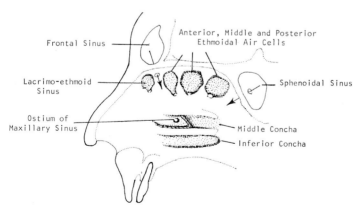

Fig. 85. Schematic view of paranasal sinuses in the adult and their communications with the nose. The middle concha has been sectioned to reveal the ostium of the unrepresented maxillary sinus.

The frontal sinuses start as furrows in the frontal recess of the middle meatus of the nasal fossa at 3–4 months i.u. but do not invade the frontal bone until the second year of life and are not visible radiographically before 6 years of age. They grow upward at an extremely variable rate until puberty. Even after puberty, all the paranasal sinuses appear to increase slowly in size into old age. Absence of development of the frontal and sphenoidal sinuses is characteristic of Down's syndrome (trisomy 21). Diminution or absence of sinuses is also found in Apert's syndrome (acrocephalo-syndactyly).

SELECTED BIBLIOGRAPHY

BLANTON, P. L., and BIGGS, N. L. (1969), 'Eighteen Hundred Years of Controversy: The Paranasal Sinuses', *Am. J. Anat.*, **124**, 135.

CULLEN, R. L., and VIDIC, B. (1972), 'The Dimensions and Shape of the Human Maxillary Sinus in the Perinatal Period', *Acta Anat.*, **83**, 411.

HAJNIŠ, K., and POZDĚNOVA, L. (1972), 'The Form, Size, and Capacity of the Frontal Sinus', *Folia Morphol. (Praha)*, **20**, 273.

KANAGASUNTHERAM, R., and RAMSBOTHAM, M. (1968), 'Development of the Human Nasopharyngeal Epithelium', *Acta Anat.*, **70**, 1.

KHOO, F. Y., KANAGASUNTHERAM, R., and CHIA, K. B. (1967), 'Variation of the Lateral Recesses of the Nasopharynx', *Archs Otolar.*, **86**, 456.

KILLEY, H. C., and KAY, L. W. (1975), *The Maxillary Sinus and its Dental Implications*. Bristol: Wright.

RITTER, F. N. (1978), *The Paranasal Sinuses*. 2nd ed. St. Louis: Mosby.

SCHAEFFER, J. P. (1920), *The Embryology, Development and Anatomy of the Nose, Paranasal Sinuses, Nasolacrimal Passageways and Olfactory Organ in Man*. Philadelphia: Blakistons.

VIDIC, B. (1971), 'The Morphogenesis of the Lateral Nasal Wall in the Early Prenatal Life of Man', *Am. J. Anat.*, **130**, 121.

CHAPTER 12

THE MANDIBLE

THE first structure to develop in the primordium of the lower jaw is the mandibular division of the trigeminal nerve that precedes the mesenchymal condensation forming the first (mandibular) branchial arch. The prior presence of the nerve has been postulated as being necessary to induce osteogenesis by the production of neurotrophic factors. The mandible is derived from ossification of an osteogenic membrane formed from ectomesenchymal condensation at 36–38 days of development. The mandibular ectomesenchyme must initially interact with the epithelium of the mandibular arch before primary ossification occurs. The resulting intramembranous bone lies lateral to Meckel's cartilage of the first

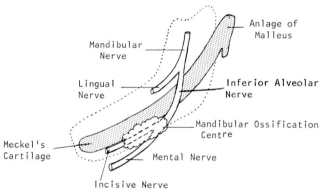

Fig. 86. Schema of centre of ossification of mandible lateral to Meckel's cartilage at the bifurcation of the inferior alveolar nerve.

(mandibular) branchial arch (p. 56) (*Fig. 86*). A single ossification centre for each half of the mandible arises in the 6th week i.u.,* in the region of the bifurcation of the inferior alveolar nerve and artery into mental and incisive branches. The ossifying membrane is located lateral to Meckel's cartilage and its accompanying neurovascular bundle. Ossification spreads from the primary centre below and around the inferior alveolar nerve and its incisive branch, and upwards to form a trough for the developing teeth. Spread of the intramembranous ossification dorsally and ventrally forms the

---

*The mandible and the clavicle are the first bones to begin to ossify.

127

body and ramus of the mandible. Meckel's cartilage becomes surrounded and invaded by bone. Ossification stops dorsally at the site that will later become the mandibular lingula, from where Meckel's cartilage continues into the middle ear. The prior presence of the neurovascular bundle ensures the formation of the mandibular foramen and canal, and the mental foramen.

The first branchial arch core of Meckel's cartilage almost meets its fellow of the opposite side ventrally. It diverges dorsally to end in the tympanic cavity of each middle ear, which is derived from the first pharyngeal pouch, and is surrounded by the forming petrous portion of the temporal bone. The dorsal end of Meckel's cartilage ossifies to form the basis of two of the auditory ossicles, viz., the malleus and incus. The third ossicle, the stapes, is derived primarily from the cartilage of the second branchial arch (Reichert's cartilage) (*see* p. 57 and p. 182).

The major portion of Meckel's cartilage disappears.* Parts of the cartilage transform into the sphenomandibular and anterior malleolar ligaments. A portion of Meckel's cartilage contributes to the formation of the spine of the sphenoid bone. A further small part of its ventral end, from the mental foramen ventrally to the symphysis, forms accessory endochondral ossicles that are incorporated into the chin region of the mandible. Meckel's cartilage dorsal to the mental foramen undergoes resorption on its lateral surface at the same time as intramembranous bony trabeculae are forming immediately lateral to the resorbing cartilage. Thus, the cartilage from the mental foramen to the lingula is not incorporated into the osseous formation of the mandible.

Secondary accessory cartilages appear between the 10th and 14th weeks i.u. to form the head of the condyle, part of the coronoid process, and the mental protuberance (*Fig. 87*). The appearance of these secondary mandibular cartilages is dissociated from the primary branchial cartilage (Meckel's) or that of the chondrocranium. The secondary cartilage of the coronoid process is believed not to be self-differentiating, but represents a developmental response following differentiation of the temporalis muscle within which the coronoid process appears. The coronoid accessory cartilage becomes incorporated into the expanding intramembranous bone of the ramus and disappears before birth. In the mental region, on either side of the symphysis, one or two small cartilages appear and ossify in the 7th month i.u. to form a variable number of *mental ossicles* in the fibrous tissue of the symphysis. The ossicles become incorporated into the intramembranous bone when the symphysis menti is

---

*Meckel's cartilage lacks the enzyme phosphatase found in ossifying cartilages, thus precluding its ossification. Meckel's cartilage does however persist until as late as the 24th week i.u. before it disappears.

converted from a syndesmosis into a synostosis during the first postnatal year.

The condylar secondary cartilage appears during the 10th week of development as a cone-shaped cartilage developing in the ramal region. This condylar cartilage is the primordium of the future condyle. Cartilage cells differentiate from its centre, and by interstitial and appositional growth, the cartilage condylar head increases in size. By the 14th week, the first evidence of endochondral bone formation appears in the condyle region. The condylar cartilage serves as an important centre of growth* for the ramus and body of the mandible. Much of the cone-shaped cartilage is replaced with bone by the middle of fetal life, but its upper end persists into adulthood, acting both as a growth cartilage and as an articular cartilage. Changes in mandibular position and form are related to the direction and amount of condylar growth. Condylar growth rate increases at puberty, peaking between $12\frac{1}{2}$ and 14 years of age. While growth at the condylar cartilage normally ceases at about the 20th year of life, the continued presence of the cartilage thereafter provides a potential for growth, which is realized in such abnormal growth conditions as acromegaly.

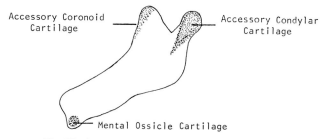

Fig. 87. Accessory cartilages of the fetal mandible.

The shape and size of the diminutive fetal mandible undergo considerable transformation during its growth and development. The ascending ramus of the neonatal mandible is low and wide; the coronoid process is relatively large and projects well above the condyle; the body is merely an open shell containing the buds and partial crowns of the deciduous teeth; the mandibular canal runs low in the body. The initial separation of the right and left bodies of the mandible at the midline symphysis menti is gradually eliminated

---

*The nature of this growth being primary, as an initial source of morphogenesis, or secondary, compensating for functional stimulation, is controversial, but experimental evidence indicates the need for mechanical stimuli for normal growth to occur.

between the 4th and 12th months postnatally, when ossification converts the syndesmosis into a synostosis, uniting the two halves.

While the mandible appears in the adult as a single bone, it is developmentally and functionally divisible into several skeletal subunits (*Fig. 88*). The 'basal bone' of the body forms one unit, to which is attached the alveolar process, the coronoid process, the angular process, the condylar process, and the chin. Each of these skeletal subunits is influenced in its growth pattern by a functional matrix that acts upon the bone. The teeth act as a functional matrix for the alveolar unit. The action of the temporalis muscle influences the coronoid process. The masseter and medial pterygoid muscles act upon the angle and ramus of the mandible, while the lateral pterygoid has some influence on the condylar process. The functioning of the related tongue and perioral muscles, and the expansion of the oral and pharyngeal cavities, provide stimuli for mandibular growth to reach its full potential. Of the facial bones, the mandible undergoes the largest amount of growth postnatally, and also exhibits the largest variability in morphology.

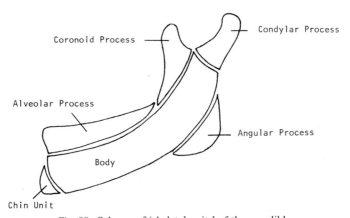

Fig. 88. Schema of 'skeletal units' of the mandible.

Limited growth takes place at the symphysis menti until fusion occurs. The main sites of postnatal mandibular growth are at the condylar cartilages, the posterior borders of the rami, and the alveolar ridges. These areas of bone deposition account grossly for increases in the height, length, and width of the mandible. However, superimposed upon this basic incremental growth are numerous regional remodelling changes, subjected to the local functional influences that involve selective resorption and displacement of the separate elements of the mandible (*Fig. 89*).

The condylar cartilage of the mandible serves the uniquely dual roles of an articular cartilage in the temporomandibular joint, characterized by a fibrocartilage surface layer, and as a growth cartilage analogous to the epiphyseal plate in a long bone, characterized by a deeper hypertrophying cartilage layer. The subarticular appositional proliferation of cartilage within the condylar head provides the basis for the growth of a medullary core of endochondral bone, on whose outer surface a cortex of intramembranous bone is laid. The growth cartilage may act as a 'functional matrix' to stretch the periosteum, thereby inducing the lengthened periosteum to form intramembranous bone beneath it. The diverse histological origins of the medulla and cortex are effaced by their fusion. The formation of bone within the condylar heads results in the mandibular rami growing in an upward and backward direction, with consequent displacement of the whole bone in an opposite downward and forward direction. Bone resorption subjacent to the condylar head accounts for the narrowed condylar neck. The attachment of the lateral pterygoid muscle to the condylar neck, and the growth and action of the tongue and masticatory muscles, are functional forces implicated in this phase of mandibular growth.

Any damage to the condylar cartilages will restrict the growth potential and normal downward and forward displacement of the mandible, unilaterally or bilaterally, according to the side(s) damaged. Lateral deviations of the mandible, and varying degrees of micrognathia and accompanying malocclusion will result.

In the infant, the condyles of the mandible are inclined almost horizontally, so that condylar growth leads to an increase in the

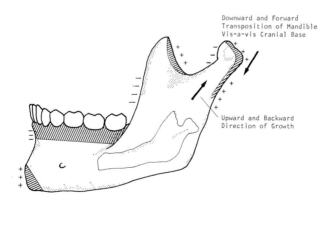

+ + +   Bone deposition
— — —   Bone resorption

Fig. 89. Schematic representation of mandibular growth with fetal mandible superimposed upon adult mandible.

131

length of the mandible, rather than increase in height. Due to the posterior divergence of the two halves of the body of the mandible (in a V shape), growth at the condylar heads of the increasingly more widely displaced rami results in an eventual total widening of the mandibular body, which, with remodelling, keeps pace with the growth in width of the cranial base (*Figs. 90, 91*). No interstitial widening of the mandible can take place at the fused symphysis menti after the first year of age, although some widening by surface apposition occurs.

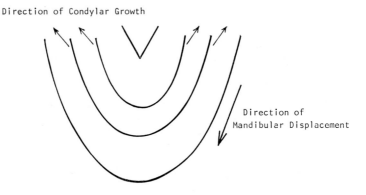

Direction of Condylar Growth

Direction of
Mandibular Displacement

Expanding V-principle accounting for
growth in width of mandible

Fig. 90. The 'expanding V' principle of mandibular growth.

Bone deposition occurs on the posterior border of the ramus, while concomitant resorption on the anterior border maintains the proportions of the ramus, and, in effect, moves the ramus backwards in relation to the body of the mandible. This deposition and resorption balance extends up to the coronoid process, involving the mandibular notch, and progressively repositions the mandibular foramen in a posterior direction, accounting for the anterior over-lying plate of the lingula. The attachment of the elevating muscles of mastication to the buccal and lingual aspects of the ramus, and to the mandibular angle and coronoid process, are influential in determining the ultimate size and proportions of these mandibular elements.

The posterior displacement of the ramus results in the conversion of former ramal bone into that of the posterior part of the body of the mandible. In this manner, the body of the mandible lengthens by the posterior molar region becoming relocated anteriorly into the premolar and canine regions. This is one of the means by which additional space is provided for the later-erupting molar teeth, all three of which initially develop in the ramus-body junction. Their forward migration, and posterior ramal displacement, both lengthen the molar region of the mandible.

Direction of Condylar Growth

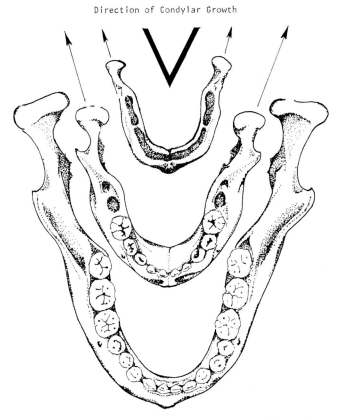

Fig. 91. Mandibles of a neonate (*top*), 4-year-old child (*middle*), and adult (*below*), illustrating the constant width of the anterior body of the mandible, but lateral expansion of their rami with growth.

The forward shift of the growing mandibular body results in the mental foramen changing its direction during infancy and childhood. The mental neurovascular bundle emanates from the mandible at right angles, or even in a slightly forward direction at birth. In adulthood the mental foramen (and its neurovascular content) is characteristically backwardly directed. This change may be ascribed

133

to the forward direction of growth that occurs in the body of the mandible, while the neurovascular bundle 'drags along' (*Fig. 92*). A contributory factor may be the differential rates of bone and periosteal growth. The latter by its firm attachment to the condyle, and its comparatively loose attachment to the body, grows more slowly than the mandibular body, which slides forward beneath the periosteum. The changing direction of the foramen has clinical implications in the administration of local anaesthetic to the mental nerve. In infancy and childhood the syringe needle may be applied at right angles to the body of the mandible to enter the mental foramen, whereas in the adult the needle has to be applied obliquely from behind to achieve entry.

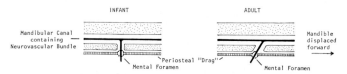

Fig. 92. Schematic explanation of the alteration of direction of the mental foramen from lateral in the infant to posterior in the adult, as a result of forward displacement of the mandible and 'dragging' of the mental neurovascular bundle.

The location of the mental foramen also alters its vertical relationship within the body of the mandible during the succession from infancy to childhood and old age. The presence of the alveolar ridge when teeth are present, whether unerupted or fully erupted, ensures the mental foramen being located midway between the upper and lower borders of the mandible. The edentulous mandible lacks an alveolar ridge, whose resorption minimizes the vertical height of the mandible. The mental foramen accordingly appears near the upper margin of the thinned mandible (*Fig. 93*).

The alveolar process develops in response to the presence of tooth buds as a protective trough, and becomes superimposed upon the 'basal bone' of the mandibular body. The alveolar bone adds to the height and thickness of the body of the mandible, and is particularly manifest as a ledge extending lingually to the ramus to accommodate the third molars. In the absence of teeth, the alveolar bone fails to develop, or resorbs in the event of tooth extraction. The orthodontic movement of teeth takes place in the labile alveolar bone, of both maxilla and mandible, and fails to involve the underlying 'basal bone'.

The chin, formed in part of the mental ossicles from accessory cartilages and the ventral end of Meckel's cartilage, is very poorly

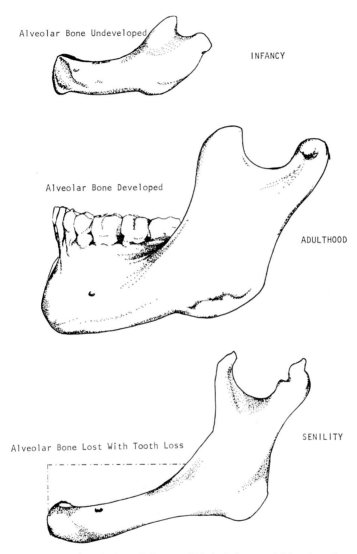

Alveolar Bone Undeveloped

INFANCY

Alveolar Bone Developed

ADULTHOOD

Alveolar Bone Lost With Tooth Loss

SENILITY

Fig. 93. Lateral view of the mandible in infancy, adulthood, and
senility, illustrating the influence of alveolar bone on the contour of
the body of the mandible. Note the altering obliquity of the angle
of the mandible. Note the stable location of the mental foramen that
appears to vary in relation to the upper border of the body of the
mandible.

developed in the infant. It develops almost as an independent sub-unit of the mandible that is influenced by sexual as well as specific genetic factors. Sex differences in the symphyseal region of the mandible are not significant in childhood, but become so with the development of other secondary sex characteristics. Accordingly, the chin becomes significant only at adolescence, and, in part, arises from development of the mental protuberance and tubercles and lingual movement of the labially inclined mandibular incisors. While small chins may be found in adults of both sexes, very large chins are characteristically found only in males. The skeletal 'unit' of the chin may in part be an expression of the functional forces exerted by the lateral pterygoid muscles that, in pulling the mandible forward, indirectly stress the mental symphyseal region by their concomitant inward pull. Bone buttressing to resist muscle stressing, that is more powerful in the male, is expressed in the more prominent male chin. The protrusive chin is a uniquely human trait that is lacking in all other primates and hominid ancestors.

The mental protuberance forms by osseous deposition during childhood. Its prominence is accentuated by the bone resorption that occurs in the alveolar region above it, creating the supramental concavity known as 'Point B' in orthodontic terminology. Under-development of the chin is known as *microgenia*.

A genetically determined exostosis that develops occasionally on the lingual aspect of the body of the mandible is known as the *torus mandibularis*. These tori are usually present bilaterally in the canine-premolar region, projecting into the oral cavity, and reach their greatest prominence in adulthood. They are unrelated to any muscle attachments, or any known functional matrices.

During fetal life the relative size of the maxilla and mandible to each other varies widely. Initially, the mandible is considerably larger than the maxilla, which predominance is later lessened by the relatively greater development of the maxilla. By about eight weeks i.u., the maxilla overlaps the mandible. The subsequent relatively greater growth of the mandible results in the upper and lower jaws being approximately of equal size by the 11th week. Mandibular growth lags relative to the maxilla between the 13th–20th weeks i.u. due to a change-over from Meckel's cartilage to condylar secondary cartilage as the main growth determiner of the lower jaw. At birth, the mandible tends to be retrognathic to the maxilla, although the two jaws may approximate each other in size. This retrognathic condition is normally corrected early in postnatal life by rapid mandibular growth and forward displacement to establish ortho-gnathia, or an Angle Class I maxillomandibular relationship. Inadequate mandibular growth would result in an Angle Class II relation, and overgrowth of the mandible would produce a Class III relation. The mandible has a capability to grow for a much longer period than the maxilla.

The mandible may be grossly deficient or absent in the condition of *agnathia*, that possibly reflects a neural crest tissue deficiency in the lower face. *Micrognathia* indicates a small mandible (*Fig. 94*). A micrognathic mandible is characteristic of a number of congenital defects, the foremost of which is the Pierre Robin syndrome. The congenitally underdeveloped mandible in this condition generally demonstrates 'catch-up' growth in the child. Other congenital facial anomalies manifesting a defective mandible are the cat-cry (*cri du chat*) syndrome, mandibulofacial dysostosis (Treacher-Collins syndrome), progeria, Down's syndrome (trisomy 21) and Turner syndrome (XO sex chromosome complement).

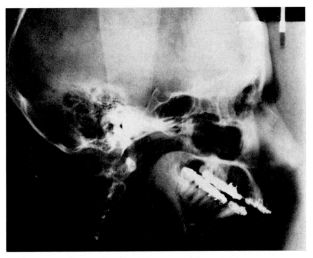

Fig. 94. Radiograph of deficient mandibular development in a 17-year-old girl. All permanent teeth are present and ortho-dontically banded. The bilaterally deficient mandibular condyles account for the symmetrical micrognathia. Maxillary dental prognathism accentuates the mandibular retrognathia. Compare and contrast with *Fig. 75*, p. 110.

The deformity of the mandible in mandibulofacial dysostosis is generally maintained throughout the growth period, whereas in instances of unilateral agenesis of the mandibular ramus, the severity of the deformity increases with age. *Macrognathia*, producing prognathism, is generally an inherited condition, but abnormal growth phenomena, such as hyperpituitarism, may also produce mandibular overgrowth of increasing severity with age.

SELECTED BIBLIOGRAPHY

BJÖRK, A. (1963), 'Variations in the Growth Pattern of the Human Mandible', *J. dent. Res.*, **42**, 400.

BURDI, A. R. (1968), 'Morphogenesis of Mandibular Dental Arch Shape in Human Embryos', *J. dent. Res.*, **47**, 50.

— — and SPYROPOULOS, M. N. (1978), 'Prenatal Growth Patterns of the Human Mandible and Masseter Muscle Complex', *Am. J. Orthod.*, **74**, 380.

EDSON PRICE, J., and ZAREM, H. A. (1979), 'Duplication of the Mandible', *Plast. and Reconstr. Surg.*, **64**, 104.

HAMPARIAN, A. M. (1973), 'Blood Supply of the Human Fetal Mandible', *Am. J. Anat.*, **136**, 67.

HERZBERG, F., and DOVITCH, V. (1968), 'Bony Trabecular Changes in the Human Mandibular Ramus from Prenatal Period to Adulthood', *Anat. Rec.*, **161**, 517.

ISRAEL, H. (1969), 'Pubertal Influence upon the Growth and Sexual Differentiation of the Human Mandible', *Archs oral Biol.*, **14**, 583.

KJAER, I. (1978), 'Histochemical and Radiological Studies of the Human Fetal Mandibular Condyle', *Scand. J. Dent. Res.*, **86**, 279.

— — (1978), 'Relation between symphyseal and condylar developmental stages in the human fetus', *Scand. J. Dent. Res.*, **86**, 500.

KNOTT, V. B. (1973), 'Growth of the Mandible Relative to a Cranial Base Line', *Angle Orthod.*, **43**, 305.

KVINNSLAND, S. (1969), 'Observations on the Early Ossification Process of the Mandible as seen in Plastic Embedded Human Embryos', *Acta odont. scand.*, **27**, 643.

— — (1971), 'The Sagittal Growth of the Lower Face during Foetal Life', *Ibid.*, **29**, 733.

LAVELLE, C. L. B., and MOORE, W. J. (1970), 'Proportionate Growth of the Human Jaws between the Fourth and Seventh Months of Intra-uterine Life', *Archs oral Biol.*, **15**, 453.

McNAMARA, J. A. (1975), (Ed.) *Determinants of Mandibular Form and Growth*. Ann Arbor: University of Michigan Center for Human Growth and Development.

MANSON, J. D. (1968), *A Comparative Study of the Postnatal Growth of the Mandible*. London: Kimpton.

MEIKLE, M. C. (1973), 'The Role of the Condyle in the Postnatal Growth of the Mandible', *Am. J. Orthod.*, **64**, 50.

MEREDITH, H. V. (1961), 'Serial Study of Change in a Mandibular Dimension during Childhood and Adolescence', *Growth*, **25**, 229.

MIETHKE, VON R. R. (1978), 'Beobachtungen zur Entwicklung vorgeburtlicher Progenion', *Fortschr. Kieferorthop.*, **39**, 444.

MONGINI, F. (1972), 'Remodelling of the Mandibular Condyle in the Adult and its Relationship to the Condition of the Dental Arches', *Acta anat.*, **82**, 437.

MOSS, M. L., and RANKOW, R. (1968), 'The Role of the Functional Matrix in Mandibular Growth', *Angle Orthod.*, **38**, 95.

Moss, M. L., and Simon, M. R. (1968), 'Growth of the Human Mandibular Angular Process: A Functional Cranial Analysis', *Am. J. phys. Anthrop.*, **28**, 127.

Petrovic, A. G. (1972), 'Mechanisms and Regulation of Mandibular Condylar Growth', *Acta morph. neerl.-scand.*, **10**, 25.

Pruzansky, S., and Richmond, J. B. (1954), 'Growth of Mandible in Infants with Micrognathia', *Am. J. dis. Child.*, **88**, 29.

Roche, A. F. (1967), 'The Elongation of the Mandible', *Am. J. Orthod.*, **53**, 79.

Yamamoto, S. (1979), 'Anatomical Studies of the Fetal Mandibular Body', *Bull. Tokyo dent. Coll.*, **20**, 37.

CHAPTER 13

THE TEMPOROMANDIBULAR JOINT

THE temporomandibular joint is a secondary development, both in its evolutionary (phylogenetic) and embryological (ontogenetic) history. The joint between the malleus and incus that develops at the dorsal end of Meckel's cartilage is phylogenetically the primary jaw joint,* and is homologous with the jaw joint of reptiles. With the development, both in evolution and embryologically, of the middle ear chamber, this primary Meckel's joint loses its association with the mandible, and reflects the adaptation of the bones of the primitive jaw joint to sound conduction (*see* Chap. 18). The mammalian temporomandibular joint develops as an entirely new and separate jaw joint mechanism.

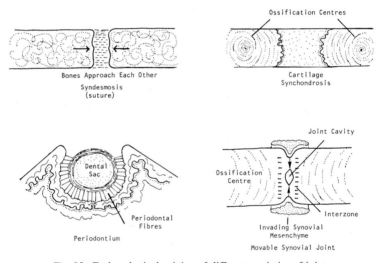

Fig. 95. Embryological origins of different varieties of joints.

The embryonic development of the temporomandibular joint differs considerably from the development of other synovial joints, reflecting its complicated evolutionary history. Most synovial joints have completed their initial cavity development by the 7th week i.u.,

*The primitive joint between Meckel's cartilage and the incus may briefly function as a jaw joint in the human embryo, since mouth-opening movements start at 8 weeks i.u., well before the definitive temporomandibular joint has developed.

140

while the temporomandibular joint has scarcely begun development at this age. Whereas limb joints develop directly into their adult form by cavity formation within the single blastema from which both adjoining endochondral bones develop (*Fig. 95*), the temporomandibular joint develops from initially widely separated temporal and condylar blastema that grow towards each other (*Fig. 96*). Further contrast with other synovial joints is evident in the presence of fibrous tissue rather than hyaline cartilage on the articular facets of the temporal mandibular fossa and mandibular condyle. In the latter site, the underlying secondary cartilage acts as a growth centre.

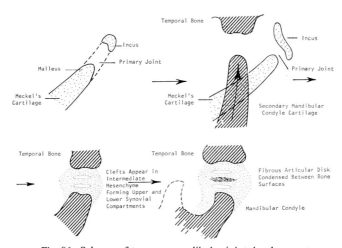

Fig. 96. Schema of temporomandibular joint development.

Between the 10th and 12th weeks i.u., the secondary cartilage of the condyle of the mandible grows towards the temporal bone, and the intervening mesenchyme differentiates into layers of fibrous tissue. During the 12th week i.u., two clefts develop in the interposed vascular fibrous connective tissue, forming the two joint cavities and thereby defining the intervening articular disk. Cavitation appears to occur prior to an invasion of synovial mesenchyme by degradation rather than by enzymatic liquefaction or cell death. Synovial membrane invasion may be necessary for cavitation to occur, but remains to be clarified. Synovial fluid production by this membrane lubricates the movements in the joint.

Muscle movement may be necessary for joint cavitation to occur. The connective tissues separating the initially discrete, small spaces, may require to be ruptured by movement for the spaces to coalesce into functional cavities. Early immobilization of developing joints

141

results in the absence of joint cavities and fusion of the articulations, with consequent skeletal distortions.

Compression of the central portion of the articular disk occurs as it assumes its characteristic biconcave shape. The tissue forming the disk is continuous with the tendon of the lateral pterygoid muscle anteriorly, and posteriorly it attaches to that portion of Meckel's cartilage which is differentiating into the malleus. This posterior extension of the disk maintains its attachment to the malleus during fetal life, the extension passing into the tympanic cavity between the petrous and tympanic ring portion of the temporal bone as the diskomalleolar ligament. At 22 weeks i.u. the petrous and tympanic ring portions of the temporal bone fuse, but the site remains identified as the petrotympanic fissure.

A condensation of mesenchyme forms the anlage of the joint capsule, progressively isolating the joint with its synovial membrane from the surrounding tissues. The joint capsule formed of fibrous tissue is present at the time of birth.

The temporomandibular joint of the newborn child is a comparatively lax structure, whose stability is solely dependent upon the capsule surrounding the joint. At birth, the mandibular fossa is practically flat, and there is no articular tubercle (*see Fig. 68*, p. 97). Only after eruption of the deciduous dentition does the articular tubercle begin to become prominent, and does not complete its development until the 12th year of life.

SELECTED BIBLIOGRAPHY

BAUME, L. J. (1962), 'Ontogenesis of the Temporomandibular Joint', *J. dent. Res.*, **41**, 1327.

— — and HOLZ, J. (1970), 'Ontogenesis of the Human Temporomandibular Joint: Development of the Temporal Components', *Ibid.*, **49**, 864.

COLEMAN, R. D. (1970), 'Temporomandibular Joint: Relation of the Retrodiskal Zone to Meckel's Cartilage and Lateral Pterygoid Muscle', *Ibid.*, **49**, 626.

FURSTMAN, L. (1963), 'The Early Development of the Human Temporomandibular Joint', *Am. J. Orthod.*, **49**, 672.

LEVY, B. M. (1964), 'Embryological Development of the Temporomandibular Joint', in *The Temporomandibular Joint* (Ed. SARNAT, B. G.), 2nd ed., Ch. 3. Springfield, Ill.: Thomas.

LINCK, G., and PORTE, A. (1978), 'Differentiation during Development of the Synovial Cavity in the Mouse', *Cell. Tiss. Res.*, **195**, 251.

MOFFETT, B. C. (1965), 'The Morphogenesis of Joints', in *Organogenesis* (Ed. DEHAAN, R. C., and URSPRUNG, H.), pp. 301–313. New York: Holt.

MURRAY, P. D. F., and DRACHMAN, D. B. (1969), 'The Role of Movement in the Development of Joints and Related Structures: The Head and Neck in the Chick Embryo', *J. Embryol. exp. Morph.*, **22,** 349.

O'RAHILLY, R. and GARDNER, E. (1978), 'The Embryology of Movable Joints' in *The Joints and Synovial Fluid*, Vol. 1. (Ed. SOKOLOFF, L.), Ch. 2. New York: Academic Press.

SYMONS, N. B. B. (1952), 'The Development of the Human Mandibular Joint', *J. Anat.*, **86,** 326.

THILANDER, B., CARLSSON, G. E., and INGERVALL, B. (1976), 'Postnatal Development of the Human Temporomandibular Joint: Histology and Microradiography, *Acta odont. scand.*, **34,** 117; 133.

VAN DONGEN, G. K. (1970), 'The Formation of the Articular Disc of the Temporomandibular Joint', *Netherlands Dent. J.*, **77,** Suppl. 5, 14.

YUODELIS, R. A. (1966), 'The Morphogenesis of the Human Temporomandibular Joint and its Associated Structures', *J. dent. Res.*, **45,** 182.

— — (1966), 'Ossification of the Human Temporomandibular Joint', *Ibid.*, **45,** 192.

CHAPTER 14

SKULL GROWTH:
SUTURES AND CEPHALOMETRICS

In cranial development, the contents induce the container ...

J. SCHOWING, 1974

THE hard unyielding nature of the bones of the skull that are studied postmortem belie the plasticity of bone tissue in the living. It is this plasticity, responsive to the influences of the surrounding soft tissues and the metabolism of the individual, that allows bone growth, and incidentally, bone distortions, to occur.

The mechanisms of bone growth have been previously described (*see* Chapter 6) and it is the purpose of this chapter to collate the growth of all the disparate components of the skull detailed in the preceding Chapters 7–13, to provide a basis for clinical analysis of the growing skull. Comparatively little attention has been directed towards prenatal *growth* of the skull, by comparison with its prenatal *development*. Most studies have been directed towards postnatal skull growth because of its clinical significance and the possibilities of therapeutic intervention in the event of abnormalities occurring.

Study of skull growth is conducted at both the macroscopic and microscopic levels of investigation. Examination of bone growth at the microscopic level involves study of osteoblastic and osteo-clastic activity, vascular alterations and correlation of patterns of lamellar organization with surface remodelling. Microradiography enables the progress of mineralization in bone trabeculae to be examined, and labelling with radioactive isotopes and intravital dyes provides information about sites of bone deposition and resorp-tion. The use of intravital bone labelling dyes enables a three-dimensional contour of a forming bone front to be marked in serial sections, thereby establishing the pattern of bone growth.

Skull growth is studied at the anatomical level by measuring overall changes in shape, size and structure using post-mortem material, and with cephalometric radiographic techniques in the living. Comparison of measurements between radiographic land-marks on skull radiographs provides a basis for assessing facial growth patterns. The measurement of distances between landmarks and the angles between skull planes constitutes *cephalometrics* employed in diagnostic orthodontic practice.

Skull growth results from a combination of: (1) bone remodelling (deposition and resorption) (*see* p. 70), (2) apposition of bone at sutures and synchondroses, and (3) transposition-displacement of enlarged and remodelled bones.

Synchondroses

Endochondral bone junctional sites are known as synchondroses where cartilage is interposed between contiguous bones. Skull growth may occur by intrinsic cartilage growth or by endochondral bone apposition. A number of synchondroses exist prenatally, most of which disappear soon after birth. The most persistent synchondrosis, of significance in postnatal skull growth, is the spheno-occipital synchondrosis (*see* p. 98). The spheno-ethmoidal junction may persist postnatally as a synchondrosis although desmolytic degeneration of the cartilage produces a suture that is of minimal significance in postnatal growth, even though fusing only late in adolescence.

A synchondrosis between condylar portions of the occipital bones may contribute slightly to skull growth and fuses between 3 and 5 years after birth (*see* p. 93). The three synchondroses between parts of the prenatal sphenoid bone (the midsphenoidal synchondrosis between the presphenoid and postsphenoid, and the bilateral synchondroses between the body and greater wings of the sphenoid) all fuse at the time of birth, and do not contribute to postnatal skull growth.

Sutures

Sutures are one of a variety of immovable bone joints (synarthroses), that, by definition, are limited to the skull. Sutures play a significant role in skull growth. While they form a firm bond between adjacent bones, sutures allow slight movement to occur, thereby absorbing mechanical stress. Intramembranous skull bones are separated by a zone of connective tissue, the sutural ligament or membrane, made up of a number of layers (*Fig. 97*). The sutural ligament is

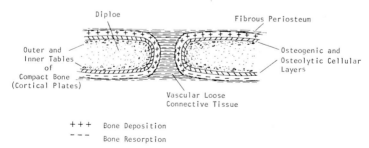

Fig. 97. Schematic diagram of suture between calvarial bones.

part of the initial membrane in which the bones ossify. The suture sites appear to inhibit osteogenesis by an as yet unknown mechanism, thus determining their location between encroaching adjacent bones. The sutures of the calvaria differ from those of the facial skeleton, reflecting the slightly different mechanisms of intramembranous osteogenesis in the two areas. The calvarial bones develop in the ectomeninx and their intervening sutures are composed of parallel fibres continuous with the pericranium and dura mater. By contrast, the facial bones ossify in relatively unstructured mesenchyme, each forming a separate periosteal fibrous covering whose fibres are tangential to the bone, with no fibres uniting adjacent bones until sutural junction is near. Secondary cartilage is a component of some sutures, most frequently in the sagittal and midpalatal sutures. This cartilage presence in membranes may be evidence of mechanical stress, as it also appears in fracture-healing sites. The possible contribution of sutural cartilages to skull growth has not been assessed.

A number of suture types are found in the skull and are described here with examples:—

1. *Serrate Suture.*—The bone edges are saw-like or notched. Examples are the sagittal and coronal sutures, that, together with the convex shape of the articulating parietal and frontal bones, enable the cranium to withstand blows of considerable force.

2. *Denticulate Suture.*—The small tooth-like projections of the articulating bones often widen toward their free ends. This union provides an even more effective interlocking than does a serrate suture. An example is the lambdoid suture.

3. *Squamous or Bevelled Suture.*—One bone overlaps another, as at the squamous suture between the temporal and parietal bones. The articulating bones are reciprocally bevelled, one internally, one externally. The bevelled surfaces may be mutually ridged or serrated.

4. *Plane or Butt-end Suture.*—The flat-end contiguous bone surfaces are usually roughened and irregular in a complementary manner. An example is the midpalatal suture.

Other types of fibrous joints found in the skull are more specialized and are not classified as sutures.

1. *Schindylesis.*—A 'tongue-in-groove' type of articulation in which a thin plate of one bone fits into a cleft in another. An example is the articulation of the perpendicular plate of the ethmoid bone with the vomer.

2. *Gomphosis.*—A 'peg-in-hole' type of articulation in which a conical process of one bone is inserted into a socket-like portion of another. An example is the initial styloid process articulation

with the petrous temporal bone, before fusion occurs. By extension, the attachment of teeth into the dental alveoli of the maxilla and mandible are described as gomphoses.

Growth at Suture Sites

Sutures are the sites of cellular proliferation and fibre formation where appositional osteogenesis contributes to the growth of the adjacent bones. Whether such growth is intrinsic and primary, causing separation of adjoining bones, or is passive and secondary to extrinsic functional matrix forces separating the bones is controversial. Experimental evidence suggests sutural bone growth is compensatory to separating forces that are the primary determinants of skull growth (*Fig. 98*).

For further discussion of this topic, *see* pp. 69 and 83.

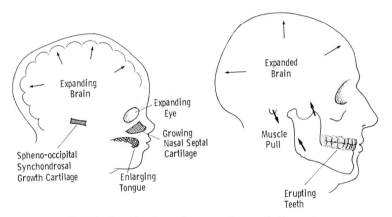

Fig. 98. Functional matrices operating on skull growth.

Sutural Fusion

The closure or fusion of sutures, by intramembranous ossification, converts the syndesmosis into a synostosis. Such fusion effectively closes off further growth potential at the suture site. Sutures begin to fuse on both the outer and inner tables of skull bones simultaneously, but closure on the outer table is slower, more variable and less complete than on the inner table. There is great variability in the timing of sutural closures, making this phenomenon an unreliable criterion of age. However, some sutures consistently close before others.

The interfrontal or metopic suture* starts closing after the first

---

*Persistence of the metopic suture into adulthood occurs in approximately 15 per cent of individuals.

year and is usually obliterated by 7 years of age, thereby converting the paired frontal bones into a single bone. The sagittal, coronal, and lambdoidal sutures fuse between 20 and 40 years of age. The occipitomastoid, sphenotemporal and squamous sutures may not be completely fused even at 70 years.

Stenosis

Premature fusion of sutures, known as *craniostenosis* or *fasciostenosis* results in premature cessation of sutural growth. Arrested bone growth occurs at right-angles to the fused suture, with consequent abnormal compensatory growth occurring in other directions, resulting in distortions of skull shape. The effects of stenosis on skull shape depend on the location of the sutures and timing of premature fusion, and may be part of a number of malformation syndromes, e.g., Apert's syndrome (acrocephalosyndactyly) and Crouzon's syndrome (craniofacial dysostosis)—(*see* p. 86). Suture closure is also sensitive to brain growth, since in microcephaly, premature closure of sutures and fontanelles occurs. Conversely, in hydrocephaly, suture fusion is delayed beyond the normal.

Isolated premature stenoses produce characteristic skull distortions. Stenosis of the sagittal suture results in an elongated, boat-shaped skull (scaphocephaly). Bilateral stenosis of the coronal sutures produces a pointed (oxycephaly), short (brachycephaly) skull. Premature stenosis of one side of the coronal suture causes obliquity of skull shape (plagiocephaly).

Premature fusion of the synchondroses of the skull base causes underdevelopment of the middle third of the face (*see* p. 100) with a reduced cranial base and excessive vaulting of the calvaria.

Cephalometrics

Study of skull growth reveals that few, if any, of the areas, points or planes that orthodontists and anthropologists use as fixed landmarks are stationary. Implanted metallic markers move during growth, by shifting with the surface to which they are attached, by being covered with new bone, or, conversely, being exposed by resorption and being freed from their site. Bone-growth markers such as metal implants, intravital staining, or radio-isotope labelling techniques give information about static areas for limited periods only during active growth.

Statistical analysis of serial radiographic measurement data by computers provides a new tool for gaining an insight into skull growth. Calculations of the mean growth patterns for large populations establish standards with which an individual child might be compared, and offers an opportunity to statistically 'predict' the growth pattern that a child might follow. Interceptive therapy

148

might be undertaken on the basis of the 'prediction' to minimize undesirable facial and dental growth patterns.

Radiographic cephalometry is now widely used clinically for analysis of craniofacial forms, allowing longitudinal growth measurements to be taken at intervals on growing children. Standardized positions of the head in cephalostats allow lateral and frontal skull radiographs of an individual to be superimposed for gathering growth data. A number of standardized radiographic landmarks and artificial planes and angles are used for cephalometric analysis. Due to growth changes, such landmarks, planes and angles are somewhat unstable and should be carefully used in analytical techniques.

The principal radiographic landmarks and their clinically recognized abbreviation in brackets are (*Figs. 99, 100*):

Nasion (N): The most depressed point of the frontonasal suture.

Anterior Nasal Spine (ANS): The most anterior point of the nasal cavity floor.

Supraspinale (Point A): The most depressed point on the concavity between the anterior nasal spine and prosthion.

Prosthion (P): The most anterior point of the maxillary alveolus.

Infradentale (I): The most anterior point of the mandibular alveolus.

Supramentale (Point B): The most depressed point on the concavity between infradentale and pogonion.

Pogonion (Pg): The most anterior point of the bony chin.

Gnathion (Gn): The point where the anterior and lower borders of the mandible meet.

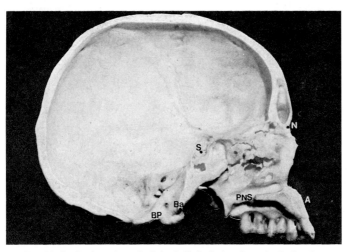

Fig. 99. Sagittal section of adult skull depicting the principal points used in cephalometrics. The abbreviations are explained in the text.

149

Menton (M): The lowest point of the mandible.

Gonion (Go): The point of intersection of the mandibular base line and posterior ramus line.

Sella (S): The midpoint of the sella turcica (pituitary fossa).

Basion (Ba): The lowermost point on the anterior margin of the foramen magnum (the posterior end of the midline cranial base.)

Orbitale (O): The lowermost point of the lower border of the orbital cavity.

Posterior Nasal Spine (PNS): The most posterior midline point of the hard palate.

Porion (Po): The midpoint of the upper margin of the external acoustic meatus.

Bolton Point (BP): The highest point of the curve between the occipital condyle and the lower border of the occipital bone.

Registration Point (R): The midpoint of the perpendicular from sella to the Bolton–nasion line.

The chief planes are:

Frankfort Plane: The line passing through porion and orbitale.

Sella–nasion Plane: The line passing through sella and nasion (SN).

Occlusal Plane: From the bisection of the upper first permanent molar (or 2nd deciduous molar) to the incisive edge of the upper central incisor.

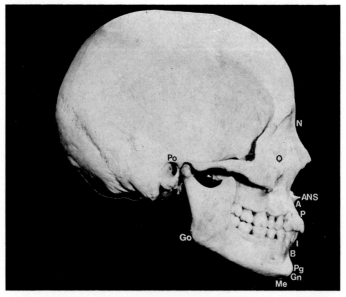

Fig. 100. Lateral view of adult skull depicting the principal points used in cephalometrics. The abbreviations are explained in the text.

Mandibular Plane: Line tangent to the lower border of the mandible passing through gnathion.

Palatal Plane: Line joining anterior and posterior nasal spines.

Facial Plane: Vertical line joining nasion to pogonion.

Bolton Plane: Line from Bolton Point to nasion.

X-Axis: Line from sella to gnathion.

Y-Axis: Line from sella to anterior nasal spine.

A number of different cephalometric analyses are available for the clinical evaluation of facial form. However, each clinician can select those linear measurements, angular measurements, and/or interrelationships that will provide the best assessment of any facial disproportions. It is the relationship of the various measurements, lines, planes, and angles that is generally more important than the absolute size of a specific measurement.

The two most frequently used angles are the SNA and the SNB angles between the sella–nasion plane and points A and B. These angles are measurements of upper and lower facial prognathism.

Certain linear measurements are very significant. The linear distance from the tip of the maxillary central incisors to NA reveals the relationship of the maxillary incisors to the NA line. The distance from the mandibular central incisors to NB relates the linear procumbency of the mandibular incisors to the NB line. These linear measurements are clinically significant as they are indicative of lip posture and aesthetics.

By utilizing the results from longitudinal growth studies, researchers

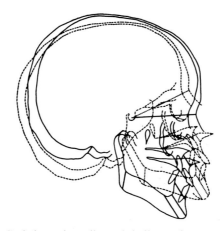

Fig. 101. Cephalometric outlines of skull growth averaged in two groups of 30 normal children from ages 4 to 17 years identified by solid lines (horizontal growth pattern) and interrupted lines (vertical growth pattern). The horizontal sella–nasion line is the basic landmark of superimposition. (*By courtesy of Dr G. W. Thompson*).

151

are attempting to develop better growth prediction methods (*Fig. 101*). This will eventually benefit the clinician who analyses facial form at the time of examination, but extrapolates beyond that to predict how the face would look at a later date with or without treatment.

SELECTED BIBLIOGRAPHY

BAUGHAN, B., and DEMIRJIAN, A. (1978), 'Sexual Dimorphism in the Growth of the Cranium', *Am. J. phys. Anthrop.*, **49**, 383.

BERKOWITZ, S. (1977), 'Orofacial Growth and Dentistry', *Cleft Palate J.*, **14**, 288.

BJÖRK, A. (1964), 'Sutural Growth of the Upper Face Studied by the Implant Method', *Acta odont. scand.*, **24**, 109.

— — (1968), 'The Use of Metallic Implants in the Study of Facial Growth in Children: Method and Application', *Am. J. Phys. Anthrop.*, **29**, 243.

— — and SKIELLER, V. (1976), 'Growth of the Maxilla in Three Dimensions as Revealed Radiographically by the Implant Method', *Br. J. Orthod.*, **4**, 53.

BROADBENT, B. H. Sr., BROADBENT, B. H. Jr., and GOLDEN, W. H. (1975), *Bolton Standards of Dentofacial Developmental Growth*, St. Louis: Mosby.

DAHLBERG, A. A., and GRABER, T. M. (Ed.) (1977), *Orofacial Growth and Development*. The Hague: Mouton Publishers.

DOBBING, J., and SANDS, J. (1978), 'Head Circumference, Biparietal Diameter and Brain Growth in Fetal and Postnatal Life', *Early Human Development*, **2**, 81.

ENLOW, D. H., et al. (1977), 'Research on Control of Craniofacial Morphogenesis', *Am. J. Orthod.*, **71**, 509.

FIELDS, H. W., METZNER, L., GAROL, J. D., and KOKICH, V. G. (1978), 'The Craniofacial Skeleton in Anencephalic Human Fetuses', *Teratology*, **17**, 57.

HARKNESS, E. M., and TROTTER, W. D. (1980), 'Growth Spurt in Rat Cranial Bases transplanted into Adult Hosts', *J. Anat.*, **131**, 39.

HERRING, S. W. (1972), 'Sutures—A Tool in Functional Cranial Analysis', *Acta anat.*, **83**, 222.

HOYTE, D. A. N. (1971), 'Mechanisms of Growth in the Cranial Vault and Base', *J. Dent. Res.*, **50**, 1447.

ISOTUPA, K. K., KOSKI, K., KOSKINEN, L., and RONNING, O. (1975), 'Experimental Studies on Craniofacial Growth', 3rd Int. Orthod. Congr. London: Crosby, Lockwood Staples.

ISRAEL, H. III (1978), 'The Fundamentals of Cranial and Facial Growth' Chap. in *Human Growth*, Vol. 2 (ed. FALKNER, F. and TANNER, J. M.) pp. 357. New York: Plenum.

JOHNSTON, L. E. (1974), 'A Cephalometric Investigation of the Sagittal Growth of the Second Trimester Fetal Face', *Anat. Rec.*, **178**, 623.

KOKICH, V. G. (1976), 'Age Changes in the Human Frontozygomatic Suture from 20 to 95 Years', *Am. J. Orthod.*, **69**, 411.

KOSKINEN, L. (1977), 'Adaptive Sutures', *Proc. Finn. Dent. Soc.* **73**, Supp. *X*, 9.

— — ISOTUPA, K., and KOSKI, K. (1976), 'A Note on Craniofacial Sutural Growth', *Am. J. phys. Anthrop.*, **45**, 511.

KVAM, E., OSTBOLL, B., and SLAGSVOLD, O. (1975), 'Growth in Width of the Frontal Bones after Fusion of the Metopic Suture', *Acta odont. scand.*, **33**, 227.

KVINNSLAND, S., and KVINNSLAND, S. (1975), 'Growth in Craniofacial Cartilages Studied by ³H-thymidine Incorporation', *Growth*, **39**, 305.

LUKE, D. A. (1976), 'Dental and Craniofacial Development in the Normal and Growth-retarded Human Fetus', *Biol. Neonate*, **29**, 171.

MCKEOWN, M. (1975), 'The Allometric Growth of the Skull', *Am. J. Orthod.*, **67**, 412.

MARKENS, I. S. (1975), 'Embryonic Development of the Coronal Suture in Man and Rat', *Acta anat.*, **93**, 257.

MAUSER, C., ENLOW, D. H., OVERMAN, D. O., and MCCAFFERTY, R. E. (1975), 'A Study of the Prenatal Growth of the Human Face and Cranium', in *Determinants of Mandibular Form and Growth*, (ed. J. A. MCNAMARA Jr). Ann Arbor: University of Michigan.

OHTSUKI, F. (1977), 'Developmental Changes of the Cranial Bone Thickness in the Human Fetal Period', *Am. J. phys. Anthrop.*, **46**, 141.

OUDHOF, H. A. J. (1978), *The Importance of the Suturae for the Growth of the Calvaria*. Thesis, University of Utrecht. (Abstract in *Netherlands Dent. J.*, **85**, Suppl. 16, 57.)

PERSSON, M. (1973), 'Structure and Growth of Facial Sutures', *Odont. Rev.* **24**, Suppl. 26, 7.

— — MAGNUSSON, B. C., and THILANDER, B. (1978), 'Sutural Closure in Rabbit and Man: a Morphological and Histochemical Study', *J. Anat.*, **125**, 313.

PRITCHARD, J. J., SCOTT, J. H., and GIRGIS, F. G. (1956), 'The Structure and Development of Cranial and Facial Sutures', *J. Anat.*, **90**, 73.

RANLY, D. M. (1980), *A Synopsis of Craniofacial Growth*. New York: Appleton Century Crofts.

RETZLAFF, E., ROPPEL, R., and MICHAEL, D. (1975), 'Possible Functional Significance of Cranial Bone Sutures', *Anat. Rec.*, **181**, 460.

— — UPLEDGER, J. E., and VREDEVOOGD., J. D. (1978), 'Cranial Suture Morphology' in *Advances in Pain Research and Therapy*, Vol. 3, New York: Raven Press.

SCHOWING, J. (1974), 'Role morphogene de l'encephale embryonnaire dans l'organogenese du crane chez l'oiseau. (The morphogenic role of the embryonic brain in the organogenesis of the cranium of the bird.) ANNEE BIOL 13 (1/2); 69–76 (In Fre. with Eng. summary) *Biological Abstracts* 58: 48213, 1974.

TEN CATE, A. R., FREEMAN, E., and DICKINSON, J. B. (1977), 'Sutural Development: Structure and its Response to Rapid Expansion', *Am. J. Orthod.*, **71**, 622.

THOMPSON, G. W., and POPOVICH, F. (1977), 'A Longitudinal Evaluation of the Burlington Growth Centre Data', *J. Dent. Res. Spec. Iss.* C 56, C71.

CHAPTER 15

THE TONGUE AND TONSILS

THE tongue arises in the ventral wall of the primitive oropharynx from the inner lining of the first four branchial arches. The covering oropharyngeal mucous membrane rises into the developing mouth as a swelling sac resulting from the invasion of muscle tissue from the occipital somites.

During the fourth week of development, paired lateral thickenings of mesenchyme appear on the internal aspect of the first branchial arches to form the *lingual swellings*. Between and behind the lingual swellings there appears a median eminence, the *tuberculum impar* (unpaired tubercle); its caudal border is marked by a blind pit, the *foramen caecum (Fig. 102)*. The foramen caecum marks the site of origin of the *thyroid diverticulum*, an endodermal duct appearing during the somite period. The diverticulum migrates caudally ventral to the pharynx to form the major portion of the thyroid gland★ *(Fig. 103)*.

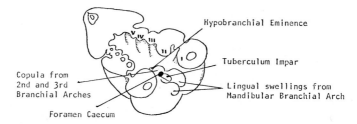

Fig. 102. Schema of tongue primordia arising in the pharynx of 4-week-old embryo. (*After Waterman and Meller.*)

The lingual swellings grow and fuse with each other, dwarfing the tuberculum impar, to provide the ectodermally derived mucosa of the body (anterior two-thirds) of the tongue.† The ventral bases of the second, third and fourth branchial arches elevate into a united, single midventral prominence known as the *copula* (a yoke). A

★Thyroid tissue occasionally remains in the substance of the tongue, giving rise to a *lingual thyroid gland*.

†It is difficult to identify the level in the adult tongue where the embryonic oropharyngeal membrane demarcated the transition from ectoderm to endoderm. It is believed that the greater part of the mucosa of the body of the tongue is of ectodermal origin.

154

posterior subdivision of this prominence is identified as the *hypo-branchial eminence*. The endodermally derived mucosa of the second to fourth branchial arches and the copula provide the covering for the root (posterior one-third) of the tongue. A V-shaped *sulcus terminalis*, whose apex is the foramen caecum, demarcates

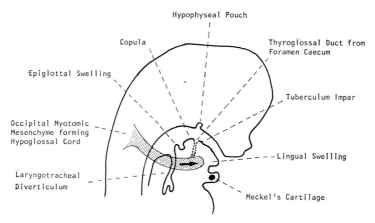

Fig. 103. Schematic midsagittal section of 5-week embryo illustrating the development of the ventral wall of the oropharynx.

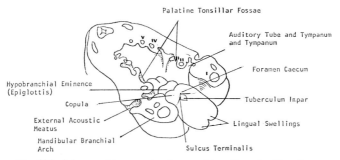

Fig. 104. Schema of tongue development in a 7-week-old embryo. (*After Waterman and Meller.*)

the mobile body of the tongue from its fixed root (*Fig. 104*). The line of the sulcus terminalis is marked by 8 to 12 large circumvallate papillae that develop at two to five months i.u. The mucosa of the dorsal surface of the body of the tongue develops fungiform papillae much earlier, at 11 weeks i.u. Filiform papillae develop later, and only develop fully post-natally. At birth, the root mucosa becomes pitted by deep crypts that develop into the lingual tonsil, the completion of which is marked by lymphocytic infiltration (*Fig. 106*).

155

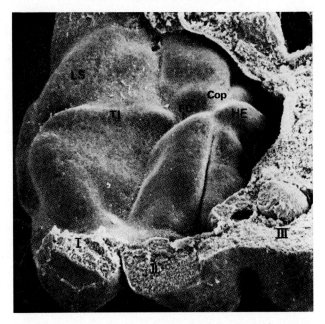

Fig. 105. Scanning electron micrograph of the developing tongue of a 33–35-day-old embryo. The branchial arches (I, II, III) border the floor of the mouth. The lingual swelling (LS) develops from the first branchial arch, the tuberculum impar (TI) between the first and second branchial arches and the hypobranchial eminence (HE) from the third branchial arch. The foramen caecum (FC) is hidden between the tuberculum impar and the copula (Cop). (*By kind permission of Drs Waterman and Meller and W. B. Saunders Co.*)

Taste buds arise by inductive interaction between epithelial cells* and invading gustatory nerve cells from the chorda tympani (facial), glossopharyngeal and vagus nerves. Taste bud formation occurs in greatest concentration on the dorsal surface of the tongue and in lesser numbers on the palatoglossal arches, the palate, the posterior surface of the epiglottis, and the posterior wall of the oropharynx. Gustatory cell formation commences as early as the 7th week i.u., but recognizable taste buds do not form until 13–15 weeks i.u., when taste perception is initiated.† Initially, only single taste buds are present in the fungiform papillae, but these multiply, possibly by branching, in later fetal life. All the taste buds in the fungiform

---

*Taste buds are derived from both ectodermal and endodermal epithelial cells.

†The addition of sacchárine to amniotic fluid has been shown to result in increased swallowing by fetuses with hydramnios (*see* footnote, p. 171).

papillae of the tongue are present at birth, but some circumvallate taste buds develop postnatally.

The muscles of the tongue arise in the floor of the pharynx in the occipital somite region opposite the origin of the hypoglossal nerve. The muscle mass pushes forward as the *hypoglossal cord* beneath the mucous layer of the tongue, carrying the hypoglossal nerve along with it (*Fig. 103*). The path of the hypoglossal nerve in the adult is explained by its embryological origins from its caudally-located brain-stem origin, tracking ventrally, superficial to the main arteries and nerves, and ending under the tongue.

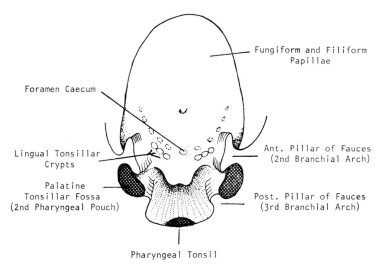

Fungiform and Filiform Papillae

Foramen Caecum

Lingual Tonsillar Crypts

Palatine Tonsillar Fossa (2nd Pharyngeal Pouch)

Ant. Pillar of Fauces (2nd Branchial Arch)

Post. Pillar of Fauces (3rd Branchial Arch)

Pharyngeal Tonsil

Fig. 106. View of the dorsum of the tongue and pharynx of the adult indicating its embryological origins. Note the 'ring' of lymphoid tissue formed by the lingual, palatine, and pharyngeal tonsils.

The combination of diverse embryological sources of the tongue is reflected in its complex innervation. The several embryological components of the tongue while moving upwards and ventrally into the mouth retain their initially established nerve supplies. Thus, the mucosal contributions of the first branchial arch (trigeminal nerve) are reflected in the lingual nerve's tactile sensory supply to the body of the tongue. The second branchial arch (facial nerve) accounts for gustatory sensation from the body of the tongue through the chorda tympani nerve.* The third and fourth arch

---

*The chorda tympani nerve is considered to be a pretrematic branch of the second branchial arch nerve (facial nerve) that invades first arch territory.

157

contributions are recognizable by the mixed tactile and gustatory glossopharyngeal and vagal nerve innervation of the mucosa of the root of the tongue. The palatoglossus muscle is innervated by the pharyngeal plexus, the fibres of which are derived from the third and fourth arch nerves. Finally, the motor innervation of all the musculature of the tongue, except palatoglossus, by the hypoglossal nerve reflects its occipital somite origin.

The rapid enlargement of the tongue relative to the space in which it develops results in the mass of the developing tongue occupying the whole of the stomodeal chamber that will later be divided up into the mouth, oropharynx, and nasopharynx. The initial partition of the stomodeal chamber, by the laterally developing palatal shelves, is delayed by the relatively enormous tongue reaching from the floor to the roof of the stomodeum. Only with later enlargement of the stomodeum does the tongue descend into the mouth chamber proper, allowing the palatal shelves to close off the mouth from the nasal fossae (p. 36).

Between birth and adulthood, the length, breadth, and thickness of the tongue normally double in dimensions. Its growth tends to be precocious relative to the size of the mouth, nearly achieving its maximum size by about 8 years of age. Such precocity is in part associated with the tongue's early role in suckling activity. The large tongue in a small mouth also accounts in part for the peculiar tongue-thrusting character of the early infantile swallowing pattern, in which the tongue fills the space between the separated jaws during swallowing. The later enlargement of the mouth facilitates the conversion to the adult pattern of swallowing, in which the tongue tip is placed against the palate behind the maxillary incisor teeth, where it remains during swallowing (*see* p. 174).

The tongue may fail to achieve a normal growth rate, resulting in an abnormally small tongue (*microglossia*) or conversely, over-development manifests as a *macroglossia*. Rarely, the tongue fails to develop (*aglossia*), or as a result of failure of fusion of its components, a forked bifid or trifid tongue may develop. Such clefts of the tongue are part of the congenital defect syndrome of orodigito-facial dysostosis, in which hyperplasia of the labial frenula and cleft palate also are manifest. Considering that the tongue influences the paths of eruption of the teeth, the state of development of the tongue is of considerable interest to the orthodontist.

The hypobranchial eminence, derived from the bases of the third and fourth branchial arches, forms the epiglottis that guards the entrance to the larynx during swallowing. During the middle of fetal life, cartilage differentiates within the epiglottis to provide it with flexible rigidity.

The sites of the second and third branchial arches in the adult pharynx are marked respectively by the anterior and posterior pillars of the fauces, between which the palatine (faucial) tonsils develop. Growth of the third and fourth branchial arches, in contributing to the root of the tongue, obliterates the ventral portions of the first and second pharyngeal pouches, leaving the dorsal portions to develop into the auditory tubes and palatine tonsillar fossae respectively (pp. 62, 63).

Tonsils

Invasion of lymphoid tissue into the palatine, posterior pharyngeal (adenoids) and lingual tonsillar regions takes place during the 3rd to 5th month i.u. These lymphoid masses encircle the oropharynx to form a ring (Waldeyer's ring) of immunodefensive tissue that grows markedly postnatally to bulge into the oropharynx (*see Fig. 106*, p. 157).

The palatine tonsils arise at the site of the second pharyngeal pouch, while the pharyngeal and lingual tonsils develop in the mucosa of the posterior wall of the pharynx and the root of the tongue respectively. Lateral extensions of the lymphoid tissue posterior to the openings of the auditory tubes form the tubal tonsils.

These disparate embryonic origins of the tonsils are reflected in differences in their cytology and in their growth and involution characteristics. Tonsillar growth is variable and cannot be considered to be true growth, but rather an individual response to the development of immunocompetence by each of the tonsils. Accordingly, the lymphoid tissue in the four tonsillar sites may not coincide in their growth and regression rates, each achieving their greatest size at different ages, and each enlarging individually in response to immunological challenges. The sizes of the tonsils are thus variable, and reflect more the state of the tonsillar immunodefence mechanisms than the age of an individual.

Lymphoid tissue characteristically grows markedly faster than other tissue systems in the body, achieving its maximum size between 8 and 12 years of age. Thereafter, lymphoid tissue rapidly regresses in size, generally being only half the size at age 20 that it was at age 10. Accordingly, the tonsils are exceedingly prominent in the 8 to 10-year-old child and, by their impingement on the nasopharyngeal airway, tend to cause mouth breathing at this age, and also possibly cause retention of the infantile pattern of swallowing. Normally, the nasopharynx enlarges in pre- and early adolescence due to concurrent accelerated growth of the bony nasopharynx and involution of the pharyngeal tonsil.

The ages between 8 and 12 years form a critical period for permanent tooth eruption. The muscle imbalances caused by mouth breathing and the infantile pattern of swallowing could adversely influence tooth eruption patterns and facial development. Dental malocclusion and a narrow 'adenoidal facies' have been attributed to mouthbreathing habits induced by exuberant pharyngeal ('adenoids') and palatine tonsillar growth. Chronic allergies producing pharyngeal mucosal hypertrophy, nasal infections, and mechanical blockage by the conchae or a deviated nasal septum may also lead to mouth breathing, producing a respiratory obstruction syndrome characterized by a tongue-thrusting swallow and dental malocclusion.

SELECTED BIBLIOGRAPHY

BAILEY, R. P., and WEISS, L. (1975), 'Ontogeny of Human Fetal Lymph Nodes', *Am. J. Anat.*, **142**, 15.

BELL, H. G., and MILLAR, R. G. (1948), 'Congenital Macroglossia', *Surgery*, **24**, 125.

BELL, R. C. (1971), 'A Child with Two Tongues (Oral-facial-digital Syndrome)', *Br. J. plastic Surg.*, **24**, 193.

BELL, W. A. (1970), 'Muscle Patterns of the Late Fetal Tongue Tip', *Angle Orthod.*, **40**, 262.

BRADLEY, R. M. (1972), 'Development of the Taste Bud and Gustatory Papillae in Human Fetuses', Chap. 6 in *Third Symposium on Oral Sensation and Perception* (Ed. BOSMA, J. F.). Springfield, Ill.: Thomas.

— — and STERN, I. B. (1967), 'The Development of the Human Taste Bud during the Foetal Period', *J. Anat.*, **101**, 743.

EL-EISHI, H. I., and STATE, F. A. (1974), 'The Role of the Nerve in the Formation and Maintenance of Taste Buds', *Acta anat.*, **89**, 599.

FARBMAN, A. I. (1971), 'Development of the Taste Bud' in *Handbook of Sensory Physiology*, Vol. IV, *Chemical Senses* (Ed. BEIDLER, L. M.). New York: Springer-Verlag.

FARMAN, A. G. (1977), 'Glossal Double Fissures in Pre- and Post-natal Human Specimens', *J. Oral Path.*, **6**, 387.

GRIFFITHS, S. J. H. (1930), 'Case of Double Tongue', *Br. J. Surg.*, **17**, 691.

HANDELMAN, C. S., and OSBORNE, G. (1976), 'Growth of the Nasopharynx and Adenoid Development from One to Eighteen Years', *Angle Orthod.*, **46**, 243.

HOLIBKA, V. (1973), 'General Laws of Development of the Lymphatic Tissue of Waldeyer's Tonsillar Ring', *Folia Morphol.* (*Praha*), **21**, 302.

HOPKIN, G. B. (1967), 'Neonatal and Adult Tongue Dimensions', *Angle Orthod.*, **37**, 132.

LEE, C. K. (1973), 'Ultrastructure of the Dorsal Lingual Epithelium in Human Embryos and Foetuses', *Archs oral Biol.*, **18**, 265.

MISTRETTA, C. M., and BRADLEY, R. M. (1977), 'Taste in Utero: Theoretical Considerations', Chap. 4 in *Taste and Development: The Genesis of Sweet Preference* (Ed. WEIFFENBACH, J. M.), DHEW Pub. No. (NIH) 77–1068, Maryland: National Institutes of Health.

PROFFIT, W. R., and MASON, R. M. (1975), 'Myofunctional Therapy for Tongue-thrusting: Background and Recommendations', *J. Am. dent. Ass.*, **90**, 403.

QUICK, C. A., and GUNDLACH, K. K. H. (1978), 'Adenoid Facies', *Laryngoscope*, **98,** 327.

SAMANT, H. C., GUPTA, O. P., BHATIA, P. L., VERMA, D. N., and RASTOGI, B. L. (1975), 'Congenital Midline Fistula of the Tongue', *Oral Surg.*, **39,** 34.

SASAKI, C. T., LEVINE, P. A., LAITMAN, J. T., and CRELIN, E. S. (1977), 'Postnatal Descent of the Epiglottis in Man', *Arch. Otolaryngol.*, **103,** 169.

SIEGEL, G. (1978), 'Description of Age-Depending Cellular Changes in the Human Tonsil', *O.R.L.* **40,** 160.

SUBTELNY, J. D. (1975), 'Effect of Diseases of Tonsils and Adenoids on Dentofacial Morphology', *Ann. Otol. Rhinol. Laryngol.*, **84,** Suppl. 19, 50.

VAN BUCHEM, F. L., and KUIJPERS, W. (1973), 'On the Origin of Lymphoid Cells in the Palatine Tonsil', *Acta Otolaryngol.*, **75,** 527.

VAN DER PUTTE, S. C. J. (1975), 'The Development of the Lymphatic System in Man', *Adv. Anat., Embryol. & Cell Biol.*, **51,** 1.

VIJ, S., and KANAGASUNTHERAM, R. (1972), 'Development of the Nerve Supply to the Human Tongue', *Acta anat.*, **81,** 466.

ZALEWSKI, A. A. (1974), 'Neuronal and Tissue Specifications Involved in Taste Bud Formation', *Ann. N.Y. Acad. Sci.*, **228,** 344.

CHAPTER 16

THE SALIVARY GLANDS

THE three major sets of salivary glands—the parotid, the submandibular, and the sublingual—originate in a uniform manner by oral epithelial buds invading the underlying mesenchyme (*Fig. 107*). All parenchymal tissue of the glands arises from proliferation of oral epithelium that may be either ectodermal (for the major glands) or endodermal (for the lingual glands) in origin. The stroma of the glands originates from mesenchyme that may be either of mesodermal or neural crest origin.

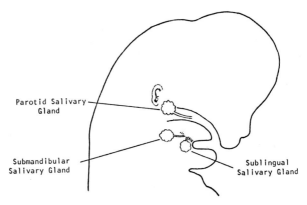

Fig. 107. Schema of the major salivary glands budding from the oral cavity. Their origins from the mouth are retained through their excretory ducts.

In all the salivary glands, following initial bud formation, there is elongation of the epithelial cell cord to form the main duct primordium. Branching from this cord produces arborization and terminal bulbs, all of which canalize to form ducts, tubules and acini. Canalization results from more rapid mitosis of the outer layers of the cord compared with the inner cell layers and from hydrostatic pressure as a result of fluid secretion by duct cells. Necrosis of cord cells has never been observed. Canalization is completed by the 6th month i.u.

The lining epithelium of the ducts, tubules and acini differentiate both morphologically and functionally. The contractile myo-epithelial cells arise from neural crest ectomesenchyme to surround the acini. Interaction between epithelia, mesenchyme, nerves and blood vessels is necessary for complete functional salivary gland morphogenesis.

The parotid gland buds are the first to appear at the 6th week i.u. on the inner cheek near the angles of the mouth, and grow back towards the ear. In the 'par-otid', or ear region, the epithelial cord of cells branches between the divisions of the facial nerve and canalizes to provide the acini and ducts of the gland. The duct and acinar system is embedded in a mesenchymal stroma that is organized into lobules and the whole gland becomes encapsulated by fibrous connective tissue. The parotid gland duct, although repositioned upwards, traces the path of the embryonic epithelial cord in the adult. An epithelial nest remnant of the parotid gland anlage that may persist in the buccotemporal space on the medial aspect of the mandible is known as the *juxta-oral organ of Chievitz*. This epithelial remnant has no known function, although it is the subject of much speculation.

The submandibular salivary gland buds appear late in the 6th week as a grouped series forming epithelial ridges on either side of the midline in the floor of the mouth at the sites of the future papillae. An epithelial cord proliferates back into the mesenchyme beneath the developing mylohyoid muscle, turning ventrally while branching and canalizing, to form the acini and duct of the submandibular gland. The mesenchymal stroma separates off the parenchymal lobules, and provides the capsule of the gland.

The sublingual glands arise in the 8th week i.u. as a series of about ten epithelial buds just lateral to the submandibular gland anlagen. These branch and canalize to provide a number of ducts opening independently beneath the tongue.

A great number of smaller salivary glands arise from the oral ectodermal and endodermal epithelium, and remain as discrete acini and ducts scattered throughout the mouth. Labial salivary glands, on the inner aspect of the lips, arise during the 9th week i.u. and are morphologically mature by the 25th week i.u.

Failure of canalization of the buds to form ducts before acinar salivary secretion commences, results in retention cysts appearing.

Agenesis of the large salivary glands is rare.

SELECTED BIBLIOGRAPHY

BERNFIELD, M. R., BANERJEE, S. D., and COHN, R. H. (1972), 'Dependence of Salivary Epithelial Morphology and Branching Morphogenesis upon Acid Mucopolysaccharide-Protein (Proteoglycan) at the Epithelial Surface', *J. Cell Biol.*, **52**, 674.

BERNFIELD, M. R., BANERJEE, S. D., and COHN, R. H. (1977), 'Basal Lamina of Embryonic Salivary Epithelia. Production by the Epithelium and Role in Maintaining Lobular Morphology', *J. Cell Biol.*, **73**, 445.

CHAUDRY, A. P., MONTES, M., and CUTLER, L. S. (1972), 'Structural and Functional Maldevelopment of Salivary Glands', in ROWE, N. H. (Ed.), *Salivary Glands and their Secretion* (Proceedings of a Symposium). Ann Arbor: University of Michigan.

CROUSE, G. S., and CUCINOTTA, A. J. (1965), 'Progressive Neuronal Differentiation in the Submandibular Ganglia of a Series of Human Fetuses', *J. Comp. Neur.*, **125**, 259.

GASSER, R. F. (1970), 'The Early Development of the Parotid Gland around the Facial Nerve and its Branches in Man', *Anat. Rec.*, **167**, 63.

GOODMAN, A. S., and STERN, I. B. (1972), 'Morphologic Development of the Human Fetal Labial Salivary Glands', *J. dent. Res.*, **51**, 990.

HAND, A. R. (1972), 'Salivary Gland Morphogenesis: Ultrastructural Criteria', in SLAVKIN, H. C. and BAVETTA, L. A. (Ed.), *Developmental Aspects of Oral Biology*. New York and London: Academic Press.

MASON, D. K., and CHISHOLM, D. M. (1975), *Salivary Glands in Health and Disease*. London & Philadelphia: W. B. Saunders.

MATSUO, Y. (1975), 'A Histological Investigation on the Developmental Process of the Submandibular and Sublingual Glands of the Human Fetuses', *J. Kyushu Dent. Soc.*, **29**, 63 (Japanese). English Abstract in *J. Kyushu Dent. Soc., Suppl.* **9**, 4.

NIELSEN, G., and WESTERGAARD, E. (1971), 'The Development of the Palatine Glands in Human Foetuses with a Crown–Rump Length of 32–145 mm.', *Acta odont. scand.*, **29**, 231.

RAMSAY, A. J. (1935), 'Persistence of the Organ of Chievitz in the Human', *Anat. Rec.*, **63**, 281.

SATOW, Y., OKAMATO, N., IKEDA, T., SHIMEDA, K., MIYABARA, S., and KAKU, E. (1969), 'Observations by Electron Microscope of the Submaxillary Glands of Human Fetuses and Newborns', *Hiroshima J. Med. Sci.*, **18** (4), 233.

SMITH, N. J. D., and SMITH, P. B. (1977), 'Congenital Absence of Major Salivary Glands', *Br. dent. J.*, **142**, 259.

SPOONER, B. S., and WESSELLS, N. K. (1972), 'An Analysis of Salivary Gland Morphogenesis: Role of Cytoplasmic Microfilaments and Microtubules', *Dev. Biol.*, **27**, 38.

THOMA, K. H. (1919), 'A Contribution to the Knowledge of the Development of the Submaxillary and Sublingual Salivary Glands in Human Embryos', *J. dent. Res.* 1(2), 95.

VOGEL, VON C., and REICHART, P. (1978), 'Aplasie der Glandulae Parotides und Submandibulares mit Atresie der Canaliculi Lacrimales', *Dtsch. zahnärztl. Z.*, **33**, 415.

YOUNG, J. A., and VAN LENNER, E. W. (1978), *The Morphology of the Salivary Glands*. London & New York: Academic Press.

CHAPTER 17

MUSCLE DEVELOPMENT

MUSCLES develop from condensations of mesodermal mesenchyme that differentiate into primitive muscle cells termed *myoblasts*. Myoblasts continue to divide until about the middle of fetal life. Myoblasts then fuse to form multinucleated *myotubes* that synthesize the contractile proteins *actin* and *myosin*. The myotubes become *muscle fibres* (*myocytes*) that initially grow by fusion of additional myoblasts. 'Myotube satellite cells' resembling Schwann cells and of possible neural crest origin are interposed between fetal myocytes to promote neural axonal growth towards differentiating, but as yet uninnervated myocytes. Neuromuscular contacts are made by most maturing myotubes, but this polyneuronal innervation is often temporary with subsequent reduction of innervation to produce variably-sized muscular motor units.

In late fetal life and postnatally, muscle growth occurs by increase in size (hypertrophy) of individual muscle-fibres, and is dependent upon the work they do.

The muscles of the head, with a few exceptions, differ in their origin from the general myotomic somite musculature of most of the rest of the body. The head muscles are derived mainly from the mesenchyme of the branchial arches (*Fig. 108*). The branchial arch mesenchyme is derived from segmental division of lateral plate mesoderm, which provides in part the lining muscle of the pharyngeal and gut wall. The branchiomeric mesenchyme of the arches gives rise to special visceral (striated) musculature, innervated by special viscero-motor cranial nerve-fibres that are under voluntary control. The transition from the specially striated visceral muscles of the mouth and pharynx to that of the 'normal' unstriated (smooth) visceral muscle of the gut takes place in the oesophagus, where voluntary control of food ingestion is lost.

The diverse craniofacial and oropharyngeal muscles may be grouped into categories corresponding to their various origins (*Fig. 109*). In migrating from their origins, the muscles carry along their initially established nerve supplies. The six extrinsic eye muscles appear to arise from three prechordal somites, the myotomes of which migrate forward to surround the eye, but retain their initial cranial nerve (III, IV, VI) connexions. The facial, masticatory and laryngopharyngeal muscles arise from the mesodermal cores of the branchial arches. A postbranchial muscle mass combines with cervical somites to give rise to the *trapezius* and *sternomastoid muscles*.

The myotomes of the occipital somites migrate ventrally as the *hypoglossal cord* to provide the muscles of the tongue (p. 157 and *Fig. 110*).

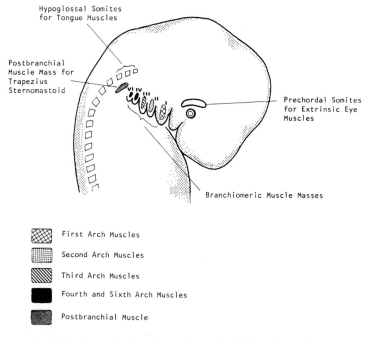

Hypoglossal Somites for Tongue Muscles

Postbranchial Muscle Mass for Trapezius Sternomastoid

Prechordal Somites for Extrinsic Eye Muscles

Branchiomeric Muscle Masses

First Arch Muscles

Second Arch Muscles

Third Arch Muscles

Fourth and Sixth Arch Muscles

Postbranchial Muscle

Fig. 108. Schematic depiction of the branchial, somite and post-branchial origins of the ocular, facial, masticatory and neck muscles prior to their migration.

The branchiomeric mesenchyme of the first branchial arch, which historically is associated with the jaws, appropriately enough gives rise primarily to the muscles of mastication and some swallowing muscles. The second arch mesenchyme★ provides the muscles of facial expression, while the branchiomeric mesenchyme of the third, fourth, and fifth or sixth arches merges into the palatofaucial, pharyngeal, and laryngeal muscle groups (for details, *see* pp. 56–58 and 117). The tongue muscles alone of those of the oropharynx are of somitic origin.

★The hyoid arch muscles, phylogenetically associated with the gill arches that regress in mammalian development, are adapted to the new mammalian function of facial expression. Fishes and reptiles have no muscles of facial expression.

166

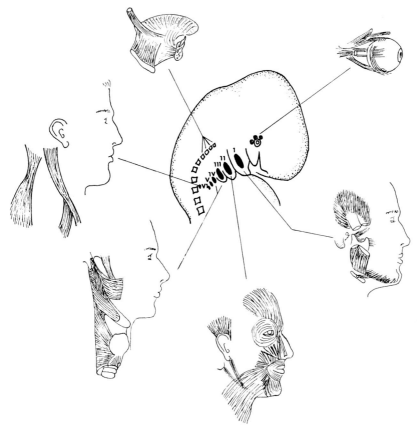

Fig. 109. Schematic description of the embryonic origins of (in clockwise order), the ocular, masticatory, facial, pharyngeal, neck and tongue muscles from presomite, postbranchial and somite sources.

The orofacial muscles are the first to develop in the body, in keeping with the cephalocaudal sequence of fetal development. The genioglossus and geniohyoid muscles are the first pre-muscle masses to differentiate from occipital and cervical myotomic mesenchyme at 32–36 days of age. The facial pre-muscle masses are formed between the ages of 8 and 9 weeks, menstrual age,★ and after migration, all of the facial muscles are present in their final positions by $14\frac{1}{2}$ weeks of age. The mylohyoid muscle and the

★Menstrual age is two weeks more than the true age (i.e., fertilization age) of the fetus. All subsequent ages mentioned in this chapter are menstrual ages (*see* footnote, p. 12).

anterior belly of the digastric which form the floor of the mouth are the earliest of the first branchial arch muscles to differentiate. The mylohyoid muscle initially attaches to the ventral border of Meckel's cartilage, but later migrates dorsally to attach to the fetal mandible.

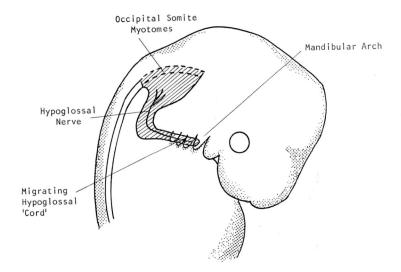

Fig. 110. Schematic depiction of the origin of the tongue muscles from the occipital somite myotomes. The path of their migration is traced out by the path of the hypoglossal nerve.

Of the palatal muscles, the tensor veli palatini is the first to develop from the first branchial arch. The levator veli palatini and palato-pharyngeus derived from the fourth and fifth branchial arches respectively next develop simultaneously. The uvular muscle develops at the time the palatal processes fuse by mesenchymal migration from the fourth branchial arch. The palatoglossus muscle, also derived from the fourth branchial arch is the last palatal muscle to differentiate.

Second arch branchiomeric mesenchyme destined to form the facial musculature is not initially subdivided into distinct muscle masses. Migration of the differentiating pre-myoblasts and early myoblasts extends from the region of the second branchial arch in sheet-like laminae. The superficial lamina spreads from a location caudal to the external acoustic meatus in all directions, and around the meatus into the temporal, occipital, cervical, and mandibular regions. Migration of the second arch branchiomeric myoblasts into the mesenchyme of the merged maxillary and mandibular processes provide the important suckling buccal and labial muscles. Differentiation of the pre-muscle masses, the development of boundaries and the gaining of attachments takes place to distinguish the delicate superficial mimetic muscles of the face. The deep mesenchymal lamina condenses to become the stapedius, posterior belly of the digastric, and stylohyoid muscles.

The masticatory muscles differentiate as individual entities from first arch branchiomeric mesenchyme, and migrate and gain attachment to their respective sites of origin on the cranium and of insertion on the mandible. The masseter and medial pterygoid have little distance to migrate, but their growth and attachments are closely associated with the mandibular ramus, which is constantly being remodelled during the early, active growth period. As a consequence, these muscles must be continually readjusting their insertions, and to a much lesser extent, their sites of origin. The insertion of the lateral pterygoid into the head and neck of the rapidly remodelling mandibular condyle requires its constant re-attachment, together with elongation concomitant with spheno-occipital synchondrosal growth, which synchondrosis intervenes between the origin and insertion of the muscle. The temporalis muscle's origin from the temporal fossa expands a considerable distance from its site of insertion as the muscle becomes employed in mastication. Its insertion, too, has to re-attach constantly to the rapidly resorbing anterior border of the ramus and coronoid process during the most active growth period. The attachments of the buccinator muscle to the maxilla and mandible also require readjusting as the alveolar processes grow.

The histogenesis and morphogenesis of muscles and nerves influence each other, and as the muscle masses form, the nerve and blood-supply to them differentiates. Nerve and vascular connexions are established at the time of muscle-fibre development, and persist even after migration of muscles away from their site of origin, which explains the long and sometimes tortuous paths that nerves and arteries may follow in adult anatomy. The wide paths of distribution of the facial nerve and the facial artery to the mimetic facial muscles serve as an example. Neuromuscular connexions are essential for full muscular development, and if they fail to occur, the muscle-fibres do not develop beyond a certain stage, and later undergo degeneration. Functional muscular activities begin as soon as neurological reflex paths are established.

Muscle-fibres gain their attachments to bone some time after their differentiation. The attachment of muscles to bones has some influence on bone formation, particularly as the muscles become functional and exert forces that invoke Wolff's Law of bone response. The hypertrophy of muscles is associated with enlargement of

169

correlated skeletal units, while the converse of muscle atrophy often induces a like response in the associated bones.

The earliest muscle movement is believed to be reflex in origin, and not any type of spontaneous activity. Muscular response to a stimulus first develops in the perioral region, as a result of tactile cutaneous stimuli applied to the lips, indicating that the trigeminal nerve is the first cranial nerve to become active.* The earliest movements in response to such exteroceptive stimuli have been elicited at $7\frac{1}{2}$ weeks' menstrual age. Spontaneous muscle movements are believed to begin only at $9\frac{1}{2}$ weeks' menstrual age. Stroking the face of the $7\frac{1}{2}$-week embryo produces a reflex bending of the head and upper trunk away from the stimulus as a total neuromuscular response. This early contralateral avoiding reaction recapitulates the phylogenetically protective reflexes of primitive creatures, to be replaced only later by a positive ipsilateral response to a stimulus.

Stimulation of the lips of the fetus at $8\frac{1}{2}$ weeks results in an incomplete but active reflex opening of the mouth in conjunction with all of the neuromuscular mechanism sufficiently mature to react at this age. From $8\frac{1}{2}$ to $9\frac{1}{2}$ weeks of age, mouth opening forms part of a total contralateral reflex response to a stimulus, with lateral head and trunk flexion, movement of the rump and all four extremities. Mouth opening without concomitant head or extremity movements can be elicited only much later at about $15\frac{1}{2}$ weeks of development. Mouth closure is initially passive, but after the 11th week it is active and rapid as a result of the initiation of muscle stretch reflex activity. Swallowing begins at $12\frac{1}{2}$ weeks in association with extension reflexes, while at 13 to 14 weeks the early activity of the facial muscles may be manifested by a sneering expression on the face of the fetus in response to eyelid stimulation. The angle of the mouth is retracted, the lateral part of the upper lip is elevated, and the ala of the nose is raised on the ipsilateral side only, and not bilaterally as occurs postnatally. These early motor capabilities are entirely unrelated to any emotions. The spread of facial muscle activity is portrayed by the ability of the fetus to squint and scowl at 15 weeks i.u. Tongue movements may begin as early as $12\frac{1}{2}$ weeks. Lip movements become active at $14\frac{1}{2}$ weeks, while the gag reflex may be elicited at $18\frac{1}{2}$ weeks.

The early differentiation of the mylohyoid and digastric muscles would account for the early mouth-opening ability, which may play a part in normal development. The withdrawal of the tongue from between the vertical palatal shelves (p. 114) and the development of synovial cavities in the temporomandibular joint (p. 141) may be dependent on these early mouth movements.

---

*Myelization, an indicator of nerve activity, appears first in the trigeminal nerve at 12 weeks, but is not completed until the second or third year after birth.

From ten weeks age onward, mouth-opening reflexes become progressively less associated with a total lateral body reflex response to a stimulus, indicating the development of inhibitory nerve pathways. However, head movements remain strongly associated with mouth movements even into the postnatal period, accounting for the 'rooting reflex', whereby perioral stimulation leads to ipsilateral head rotation, which is associated with suckling in the infant. Remnants of the total reflex response are further seen in the hand grasp reflex noticeable when an infant suckles.

Complex suckling movements involving mouth opening, lip protrusion, and tongue movements are not manifested spontaneously until 24 weeks of age, although individual components of the total movement may be elicited by stimulation about the mouth much earlier. Intra-uterine thumb sucking has been demonstrated as early as 18 weeks. Crying may start between the 21st and 29th weeks i.u., reflecting the related muscle activities of the larynx and spasmodic 'inhalation' and 'exhalation' by the thoracic cage musculature. Full swallowing and suckling permitting survival occurs at only 32–36 weeks of fetal age. Some preliminary earlier swallowing occurs as early as 12 weeks, when the fetus literally drinks the amniotic fluid in which it is bathed.* The co-ordinated effective combination of suckling and swallowing is an indicator of neurological maturation that is particularly important for the survival of premature infants. Respiratory movements may be elicited by stimulus as early as 13 weeks, but spontaneous rhythmical respiration necessary for survival does not occur until very much later. Increasingly complex muscle movements, producing mastication and speech, are dependent upon the development of the appropriate reflex proprioceptive mechanisms.

The cutaneous covering of the lips of the fetus is sharply delineated from the adjacent skin and oral mucosa (*Fig. 111*). The primitive epithelium of the vermilion surface of the lip forms a distinctive multilayered periderm that is later shed in utero. At birth, the surface of the infant's lips (*Fig. 112*) is subdivided into a central highly mobile suckling area characterized by fine villi—*pars villosa*, distinct from an outer smooth zone—*pars glabra* and an inner vestibular zone—*pars mucosa*. The villous portion of the infant lip is adhesive—more so than the glabrous or vestibular portions—

---

*The importance of this early swallowing is indicated by the excess amount of amniotic fluid (hydramnios) found in the amniotic sacs of fetuses unable to swallow because of oesophageal atresia. Near term, the normal fetus will swallow as much as 750 ml. of amniotic fluid a day. The swallowed amniotic fluid is absorbed by the gut, whence it is carried by the fetal blood-stream to the placenta. It is then passed on to the maternal blood for elimination. Interestingly, amniotic fluid is not normally inspired into the lungs of the fetus.

that may result from the blood-vessels in the villi swelling during suckling, establishing an airtight seal around the nipple.

The conspicuous philtrum of the neonatal upper lip gradually loses its clarity during childhood as the central depression becomes shallower in the adult. The rare phenomenon of *double lip* (either upper or lower) results from hypertrophy of the inner pars villosa and an exaggerated boundary line demarcating it from the outer pars glabra. *Congenital fistulae* of the lower lip, usually bilateral, seldom unilateral and occasionally median may occur rarely. Their aetiology is obscure.

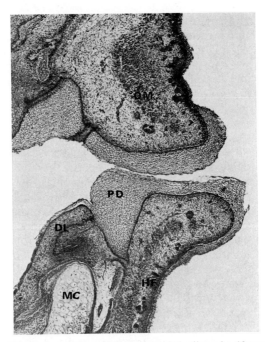

Fig. 111. Paramedian sagittal section of the lips of a 12-week-old fetus. Note the nature of the multilayered periderm (PD), the developing orbicularis oris muscle (OM), the dental lamina (DL) and Meckel's cartilage (MC). Hair follicles (HF) are forming in the cutaneous areas. (×56.) (*By courtesy of Dr R. R. Miethke.*)

With use, muscles increase in size due to the hypertrophy of individual fibres. The converse, muscle disuse, results in their atrophy. At birth, the suckling muscles of the lips (orbicularis oris) and cheeks (buccinators) are relatively better developed than the muscles of mastication (*Fig. 113*). Indeed, at birth the mobility of the face is

172

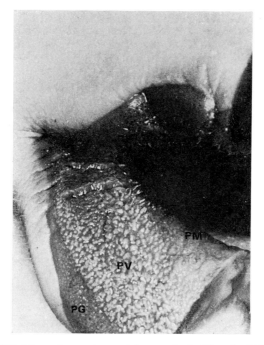

Fig. 112. Lips and commissure of the mouth of a 39-week-old fetus. Note in the lower lip the outermost smooth *pars glabra* (PG) that narrows towards the commissure. The central *pars villosa* (PV) is covered with fine villi. The inner vestibular zone, *pars mucosa* (PM) is continuous with the vestibule of the mouth. (approx. ×4.) (*By courtesy of Dr R. R. Miethke.*)

limited to eyelids and central portions of the lips, except for some slight corrugation in the forehead and mental protuberance areas. Between birth and adulthood, the facial muscles increase four times in weight, while the muscles of mastication increase seven times in weight. The masseter and medial pterygoid are better developed at birth than the temporalis and lateral pterygoid muscles. The buccinator muscle is prominent in the cheek of the neonate. Its powerful suckling capabilities are enhanced by a large subcutaneous adipose mass, forming a 'sucking pad'★ that prevents collapse of the cheeks during suckling. The tongue musculature is well developed at birth, and the tongue shows a wide range of movement.

All the complex interrelated orofacial movements of suckling,

---

★The buccal fat pad of Bichat is peculiarly loose in texture and is bounded by a connective tissue capsule. The fat in the pad persists even in emaciation, indicating its structural and mechanical function, rather than fat storage.

swallowing, breathing and gagging are reflex in origin rather than learned, and constitute *unconditioned congenital reflexes* necessary for survival. *Conditioned acquired reflexes* develop with maturation of the neuromuscular apparatus and are generally learned as 'habits'. The development of abnormal patterns of movement ('bad habits'), is likely to be the result of conditioned fetal reflex activity developing out of sequence, or the omission of a specific response to a sequential triggering stimulus.

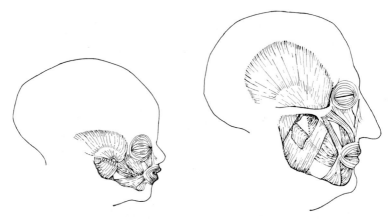

Fig. 113. Muscle development at birth and in adulthood. In infancy, the suckling facial muscles are relatively better developed than the muscles of mastication. In adulthood, the muscles of mastication are more strongly developed than the facial muscles. Compare the area of attachment of the temporalis muscle in the infant and the adult.

Prior to the eruption of the primary first molars, the infant swallows with the jaws separated and the tongue thrust forward, using predominantly the facial muscles (orbicularis oris and buccinators), innervated by the facial nerve. This pattern is known as the infantile swallow, and is a non-conditioned congenital reflex. The lips are actively sucking during swallowing, and contrary to that in the adult swallowing pattern, their action is more prominent than are the tongue movements. After eruption of the posterior primary teeth, at 18 months of age onwards, the child tends to swallow with the teeth brought together by masticatory muscle action, without a tongue thrust. This mature swallow is an acquired conditioned reflex, and is intermingled with the infantile swallow during a transition period. As the child grows older, variability of the swallowing pattern decreases as the adult swallowing pattern is

174

increasingly adopted. The movements of the mature swallow are primarily of those muscles innervated by the trigeminal nerve, viz., the muscles of mastication and the mylohyoid. Once the facial nerve musculature has been relieved of its initial swallowing duties, it is better able to perform the delicate mimetic activities of facial expression and speech that are acquired from 18 months onward.

The infant's cry is a non-conditioned reflex, which accounts for its lack of individual character and its sporadic nature. Speech, on the other hand, is a conditioned reflex, which differs among individuals, but is regular by virtue of the sophisticated control required.

Mastication is a conditioned reflex, learned by initially irregular, and poorly co-ordinated, chewing movements.* The proprioceptive responses of the temporomandibular joint and the periodontal ligaments of the erupting dentition establish a stabilized chewing pattern alined to the individual's dental intercuspation.

The conversion of the infantile swallow into the mature swallow, of infantile suckling into mastication, and of infant crying into speech, are all examples of the substitution of conditioned reflexes acquired with maturation for the unconditioned congenital reflexes of the neonate. Superimposed upon these reflex movements are voluntary activities under conscious control that are acquired by learning and experience.

The maturation of normal neuromuscular reflexes and the development of a proper equilibrium of muscular forces during orofacial growth is necessary for the production of normal jaw morphology and dental occlusion. Tongue movements and lip and cheek pressures guide erupting teeth into normal occlusion. The retention of the tooth-apart, tongue-thrusting infantile pattern of swallowing into childhood creates abnormal myofunctional pressures upon the teeth resulting in a characteristic 'open bite' pattern of malocclusion. Muscle malfunctioning, either by their hyper- or hypotonicity, particularly of the orbicularis oris–buccinator–tongue complex will result in dental malocclusion.† The pressures exerted by these muscles determine in part the form of the dental arches.

---

*The number of proprioceptive neuromuscular spindles in the lateral pterygoid muscle is much fewer than in the other masticatory muscles, accounting for its uncoordinated behaviour.

†*The ornithologist is quite absurd*
  To think a swallow is a bird;
  The swallow is a tongue-confusion,
  That causes dental malocclusion.

H. BLOOMER (1963)

SELECTED BIBLIOGRAPHY

BARNWELL, Y. M. (1977), 'The Morphology of Musculus Styloglossus in Fifteen Week Human Fetuses', *Internat. J. Oral Myol.*, **3**, 8.

— —, LANGDON, H. L., and KLUBER, K. (1978), 'The Anatomy of the Intrinsic Musculature of the Tongue in the Early Human Fetus', *Ibid.*, **4**, 5.

BLOOMER, H. H. (1963), 'Speech Defects in Relation to Orthodontics', *Am. J. Orthod.*, **49**, 920.

BOSMA, J. F. (1970), (Ed.) *Second Symposium on Oral Sensation and Perception*. Springfield, Ill.: Thomas.

— — (1972), (Ed.) *Third Symposium on Oral Sensation and Perception*. Springfield, Ill.: Thomas.

— — (1973), (Ed.) *Fourth Symposium on Oral Sensation and Perception*. Washington: U.S. Government Printing Office. DHEW Publication No. (NIH) 73–546.

BURDI, A. R., and SPYROPOULOS, M. N. (1978), 'Prenatal Growth Patterns of the Human Mandible and Masseter Muscle Complex', *Am. J. Orthod.*, **74**, 380.

BURLEIGH, I. G. (1974), 'On the Cellular Regulation of Growth and Development in Skeletal Muscle', *Biol. Rev.*, **49**, 267.

CALNAN, J. (1952), 'Congenital Double Lip: Record of a Case with a Note on the Embryology', *Br. J. Plast. Surg.*, **5**, 196.

COX, R. L. (1970), *Muscular Development and Maturation of the Dento-facial Complex: Normal and Abnormal*. Proceedings of the Workshop on Speech and the Dentofacial Complex: The State of the Art. Report No. 5. Washington: American Speech and Hearing Association.

DOMÉNECH-RATTO, G. (1977), 'Development and Peripheral Innervation of the Palatal Muscles', *Acta anat.*, **97**, 4.

GAMBLE, H. J., FENTON, J., and ALLSOP, G. (1978), 'Electron Microscopic Observations on Human Fetal Striated Muscle', *J. Anat.*, **126**, 567.

GASSER, R. F. (1967), 'Development of the Facial Muscles in Man', *Am. J. Anat.*, **120**, 357.

HANSON, M. L., and COHEN, M. S. (1973), 'Effects of Form and Function on Swallowing and the Developing Dentition', *Am. J. Orthod.*, **64**, 63.

HAZELTON, R. D. (1969), 'Origin and Migration of Facial Muscle Primordia and their Significance in Development of the Cranial Nervous System', *J. Can. dent. Ass.*, **35**, 271.

HUMPHREY, T. (1968), 'The Development of the Mouth Opening and Related Reflexes involving the Oral Area of Human Fetuses', *Ala. J. med. Sci.*, **5**, 126.

— — (1969), 'The Relation between Human Fetal Mouth Opening Reflexes and Closure of the Palate', *Am. J. Anat.*, **125**, 317.

— — (1971), *Human Prenatal Activity Sequences in the Facial Region and Their Relationship to Postnatal Development*. Proceedings of the Conference on Patterns of Orofacial Growth and Development. Report No. 6. Washington: American Speech and Hearing Association.

— — (1971), 'Development of Oral and Facial Motor Mechanisms in Human Fetuses and their Relation to Craniofacial Growth', *J. dent. Res.*, **50**, 1428.

KELLY, A. M., and RUBINSTEIN, N. A. (1980), 'Why are Fetal Muscles Slow?', *Nature*, **288**, 266.

MIETHKE, R. R. (1977), 'Zur Anatomie der Ober- und Unterlippe zwischen dem 4 intrauterinen Monat und der Geburt', *Gegenbaurs morph. Jahrb.*, **123**, 424.

MOYERS, R. E. (1964), 'The Infantile Swallow', *Rep. Congr., Eur. orthodont. Soc.*, **40**, 180.

— — (1971), *Postnatal Development of the Orofacial Musculature*, Proceedings of the Conference on Patterns of Orofacial Growth and Development. Report No. 6. Washington: American Speech and Hearing Association.

OGG, L. H. (1975), 'Oral and Pharyngeal Development and Evaluation', *J. Am. Phys. Ther. Assoc.*, **55**, 235.

ROOD, S. R. (1973), 'The Morphology of M. tensor veli palatini in the 5 mo. Human Fetus', *Am. J. Anat.*, **138**, 191.

SOENTGEN, M. L., PIERCE, L., and BRENMAN, H. S. (1969), 'Mouthing Activities in the Human Neonatal Sucking Act', *Archs oral Biol.*, **14**, 1159.

SPYROPOULOS, M. N. (1977), 'The Morphogenetic Relationship of the Temporal Muscle to the Coronoid Process in Human Embryos and Fetuses', *Am. J. Anat.*, **150**, 395.

VAN WYK, C. W. (1975), 'The Development of the Epithelium of the Junction between the Skin and the Vermilion Border of the Lip', *J. Dent. Ass. S. Afr.*, **30**, 557.

WARBRICK, J. G., McINTYRE, J. R., and FERGUSON, A. G. (1952), 'Remarks on the Aetiology of Congenital Bilateral Fistulae of the Lower Lip', *Br. J. Plast. Surg.*, **4**, 254.

CHAPTER 18

SPECIAL SENSE ORGANS

THE organs of the special senses of olfaction, gustation, vision, balance and hearing are all located in the craniofacial complex. Parts of these special sense organs initially arise in a rather similar manner.* Localized areas of surface ectoderm are induced by underlying cranial nerve extensions to thicken and differentiate into distinct *placodes*. The subsequent fates of the olfactory, lens and otic placodes will be briefly described individually.

The Nose

Development of the external apparatus of the nose has been considered together with the development of the face (p. 32).

The special sensory olfactory epithelium of the nose appears on the infero-lateral aspects of the frontonasal process towards the end of the somite period as the *olfactory (nasal) placodes (Fig. 25, p. 34)*. The relative 'sinking' of the olfactory placodes into the depths of the olfactory pits causes the specialized sensory olfactory epithelium of each placode to be ultimately located in the lateral walls of the upper fifth of each nasal cavity. The olfactory nerve cells connect with the olfactory bulb of the brain through the cribriform plate of the ethmoid bone.

The Eye

The eye is derived from surface ectoderm, neural ectoderm, neural crest tissue and mesoderm. The light-sensitive portion of the eye, the retina, is a direct outgrowth from the forebrain, projecting bilaterally as the *optic vesicles* that are connected to the brain by the optic stalks (*Fig. 114*). The presence of the neuroectodermal optic vesicles induces the overlying surface ectoderm to thicken and form the *lens placodes*. Each lens placode invaginates in its centre by the development of peripheral folds that fuse to convert the placodes into closed *lens vesicles* that sink beneath the surface ectoderm. The initially hollow lens vesicles become filled with lens fibres to form the lenses. The optic vesicles also invaginate partially to form the double-layered *optic cups*, while the optic stalks become the *optic nerves*. The outer layer of the optic cup acquires neural crest pigmentation to become the pigmented layer of the retina, while the inner layer differentiates into the light-sensitive nervous layer.

Meningeal ectomesenchyme (of neural crest origin) surrounding

---

*The organs of the special sense of gustation, the taste buds, dealt with on p. 156, differ in this respect in their origin from the other special sense organs.

the optic cups and lenses forms the *sclera* and *choroid* over the cups, the *ciliary bodies* at the margins of the cups, and the *cornea* over the lenses. Mesoderm invades the optic cups to form the *vitreous* body. The extrinsic muscles of the eye are derived from the prechordal somites (p. 166).

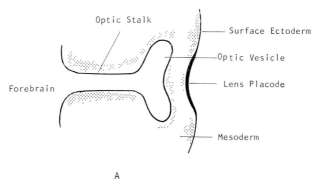

A

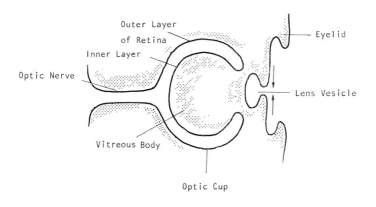

B

Fig. 114. Schematic representation of eye development. A, Optic vesicle evaginating from forebrain. B, Formation of the optic cup and lens vesicle.

The cutaneous ectoderm overlying the cornea forms the *conjunctiva*. Ectodermal folds develop above and below the cornea, and with their central core of mesenchyme, form the *eyelids*. The eyelids close at the end of the 8th week and remain closed until the 7th month i.u.

The eyes normally 'migrate' from their initially lateral positions towards the midline of the face, and over- and under-migration produce anomalies of facial appearance (*see* pp. 36, 45).

179

The Ear

The three parts of the ear—external, middle and internal—arise from quite separate and diverse embryonic origins, reflecting the complicated phylogenetic history of the adaptation of the primitive branchial arch apparatus for hearing and balance.

The external ear forms around the first branchial groove (*Fig. 48*, p. 61) that deepens to become the external acoustic meatus initially located in the mandibulo-cervical region. The auricle develops as a series of six swellings or hillocks surrounding the dorsal aspect of the first branchial groove. Three of the hillocks develop from the first (mandibular) branchial arch; the remaining three arise from the second (hyoid) branchial arch (*Fig. 115*). Differential growth

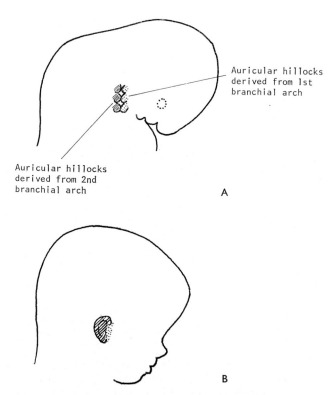

Auricular hillocks
derived from 1st
branchial arch

Auricular hillocks
derived from 2nd
branchial arch

A

B

Fig. 115. Schematic representation of the development of the auricle. A, The six auricular hillocks (three from each of first and second branchial arches) surrounding the first branchial groove (external acoustic meatus). B, The small proportion of the anterior auricle derived from the first branchial arch (dots) contrasted with the large proportion derived from the second branchial arch (slanted lines).

and fusion of the hillocks by the end of the 8th week produces the characteristic shape of the auricle. The auricle and external acoustic meatus migrate cranially from their original cervical location, and by the 4th month i.u. reach their 'normal' position. Elastic cartilage differentiates in the mesenchyme around the external acoustic meatus.

The tympanic ring of the temporal bone forms the boundaries of the tympanic membrane that closes off the external acoustic meatus from the middle ear (*Fig. 116*). The external acoustic meatus is of shallow depth in the newborn, resulting in the tympanic ring and tympanic membrane being superficially located in the neonate. At birth, the tympanic ring and membrane are markedly oblique in inclination, which orientation allows these structures that have achieved adult size by birth to be accommodated in the late fetus and infant. Outward growth of the bony tympanic ring and cartilage of the meatus deepens the meatus during infancy and childhood, and allows adult orientation of the tympanic membrane and consequently of the os icular chain.

The middle ear develops from the tubo-tympanic recess derived from the first pharyngeal pouch (p. 62). The endodermal lining of the tympanic recess comes into proximity with the ectodermal lining of the external acoustic meatus and, with a thin layer of intermediate mesoderm, forms the tympanic membrane. Expansion of the

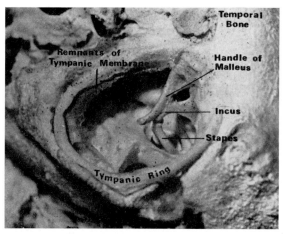

Fig. 116. Photograph of the tympanum in a neonatal skull. The tympanic membrane has been torn away to reveal the three ear ossicles *in situ*. The base of the stapes is in the fenestra vestibuli, and half the fenestra cochleae is seen below it. Note the superficial location of the middle ear in the skull of the newborn, due to the absence of a bony external acoustic meatus.

CRANIOFACIAL EMBRYOLOGY

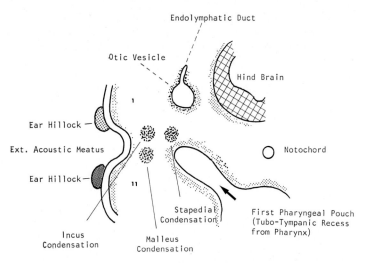

Endolymphatic Duct

Otic Vesicle

Hind Brain

Ear Hillock

Ext. Acoustic Meatus

Notochord

Ear Hillock

Stapedial
Condensation

First Pharyngeal Pouch
(Tubo-Tympanic Recess
from Pharynx)

Incus
Condensation

Malleus
Condensation

Fig. 117. Schematic illustration of the early stages (at 5 weeks i.u.) of ear development. The external ear (auricle and external acoustic meatus) is forming around the first branchial groove. The middle ear is developing from the first pharyngeal pouch and ear ossicle formation from the first (malleus, incus) and second (stapes) branchial arches. The inner ear is developing from the otic vesicle.

tympanic cavity surrounds and envelops the chain of three ear ossicles developing from the first and second branchial arch cartilages (*see* Chapter 4 and *Figs. 47, 117, 118*). The ossicles thus appear to lie within the tympanic cavity, although in reality they are outside it, separated from it by the pharyngeal endodermal membrane. The tympanic cavity achieves its ultimate adult size by 37 weeks i.u. Further expansion of the tympanic cavity postnatally gives rise to the mastoid air cells.

The auditory tube opens at birth, or is cleared of fluid by respiration. Swallowing aids the establishment of hearing that is normally impaired for the first two days after birth.

The malleus and incus* are derived from the dorsal end of the first branchial arch cartilage (*see* p. 56), the joint between them representing the primitive jaw joint (*see* Chapter 13, p. 182). The stapes is derived in part from the dorsal end of the second arch cartilage in which three ossification centres appear. The ossification†

*The incus arises from the separated end of Meckel's cartilage that corresponds with the pterygo-quadrate cartilage of inframammalian vertebrates.
†Ossification of these bones is endochondral, but the anterior process of the malleus forms independently in membrane bone. After birth, this anterior mallar process shrinks to less than one-third of its excessive length.

of the ear ossicles begins in the 4th month i.u. and proceeds rapidly to form adult-size bones by the 25th week i.u. They are the first bones in the body to attain their ultimate size. The cartilage of the otic capsule breaks down around the footplate of the stapes to form the oval window. Failure of this chondrolysis to occur is a source of one form of congenital deafness.

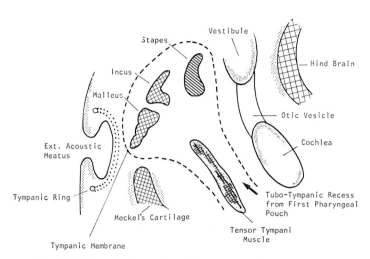

Fig. 118. Schematic illustration of later stages of ear development. The external acoustic meatus is partially surrounded by the bony tympanic ring to which the tympanic membrane is attached. The ear ossicles are enveloped by the tubo-tympanic recess, and the inner ear has subdivided into the organ of balance (vestibule) and hearing (cochlea).

The tensor tympani muscle, attaching to the malleus, is derived from the first branchial arch and is innervated by the mandibular division of the trigeminal nerve of that arch. The stapedius muscle, attached to the stapes, is derived from the second branchial arch and, accordingly, is innervated by the facial nerve of that arch.

The inner ear arises from the *otic placode* at 21–24 days i.u. and is initiated by vestibulo-cochlear nerve induction of surface ectoderm. Invagination of the placode and the apposition of its folded margins forms the *otic vesicle* or *otocyst* that sinks beneath the surface ectoderm (*Fig. 117*). Subsequent complicated configurations of the otocyst give rise to the endolymphatic duct and sac, the saccule and utricle, the three semicircular canals and the cochlear duct that together form the *membranous labyrinth*. The surrounding cartilage of the otic capsule conforms to the intricate shape of the membranous labyrinth and forms the *bony labyrinth* when intra-membranous ossification of the modiolus occurs. The rigidity imparted by the location of the labyrinths deeply embedded within bone determines a fixed orientation of the three semi-circular canals on each side to each other and also to the head, allowing for balance and centrifugal senses to be developed. The capacity of the cochlea to respond to vibratory stimuli is first established at 26 weeks i.u.

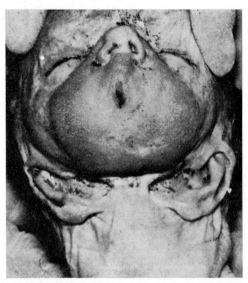

Fig. 119. A stillborn female 33-week fetus with microstomia, aglossia, agnathia, and synotia (otocephalic monster) resulting from aplasia of the first and second branchial arches. (*By courtesy of Dr G. B. Leckie.*)

Anomalies of the ear include *microtia* that afflicts the auricle, which is reduced or absent, together with a blind external acoustic meatus. Hypoplasia of the auditory tube occurs in nearly all cleft palate patients. A more severe facial anomaly is *synotia*, where the ears are abnormally located ventrally in the upper part of the neck (*Fig. 119*). The latter condition is usually associated with *agnathia* (p. 137), and the two concomitant anomalies have been attributed to an absence of neural crest tissue that normally migrates into the lower anterior face. Not only does the mandible fail to form, but the otocysts that form the ear occupy a position that would other-wise have been occupied by mandibular neural crest ectomesen-chyme. The presence and growth of the mandible appears to be a factor in determining the location of the ears.

SELECTED BIBLIOGRAPHY

ANDERSEN, H., MATTHIESSEN, M. E., and JORGENSEN, M. B. (1969), 'The Growth of the Otic Cavities in the Human Foetus', *Acta Otolaryngol.*, **68**, 243.

ANSON, B. J., and BAST, T. H. (1946), 'The Development of the Auditory Ossicles and Associated Structures in Man', *Ann. Otol. Rhinol. Laryngol.*, **55**, 467.

ANSON, B. J., and DONALDSON, J. A. (1981), *Surgical Anatomy of the Temporal Bone*, 3rd ed. Philadelphia: W. B. Saunders.

BARBER, A. N. (1955), *Embryology of the Human Eye*. St. Louis: Mosby.

BOLLOBÁS, B., and HAJDU, I. (1975), 'The Development of the Tympanic Sinus', *ORL*, **37**, 97.

BOWDEN, R. E. M. (1977), 'Development of the Middle and External Ear in Man', *Proc. roy. Soc. Med.*, **70**, 807.

GILBERT, P. W. (1957), 'The Origin and Development of the Human Extrinsic Ocular Muscles', *Contrib. Embryol. Carnegie Instn*, **36**, 59.

GORLIN, R. J. (Ed.) (1980), *Morphogenesis and Malformation of the Ear*. New York: Alan R. Liss Inc.

HANSON, J. R., ANSON, B. J., and STRICKLAND, E. M. (1962), 'Branchial Sources of the Auditory Ossicles in Man', *Arch. Otolaryngol.*, **76**, 200.

JARVIS, J. F. (1972), 'Congenital and Hereditary Abnormalities of the Ear', *S. Afr. Med. J.*, **46**, 539.

KOORNNEEF, L. (1976), 'Development of the Connective Tissue in the Human Orbit', *Acta morph., neerl.-scand.*, **14**, 263.

LAPAYOWKER, M. S. (1974), 'Congenital Anomalies of the Middle Ear', *Radiol. Clin. N. Am.*, **12**, 463.

LECKIE, G. B. (1975), 'Aplasia of the First and Second Branchial Arches', *J. Laryngol. & Otol.*, **89**, 1263.

LOPASHOV, G. V., and STROEVA, O. G. (1964), *Development of the Eye*. Jerusalem: Israel Programme for Scientific Translations.

MANN, IDA C. (1964), *The Development of the Human Eye*, 3rd ed. London: British Medical Association.

MELNICK, M., and MYRIANTHOPOULOS, N. C. (1979), *External Ear Malformations: Epidemiology, Genetics and Natural History*. Birth Defects: Original Article Series, Vol. XV, No. 9. New York: Alan R. Liss Inc.

O'RAHILLY, R. (1963), 'The Early Development of the Otic Vesicle in Staged Human Embryos', *J. Embryol. Exp. Morphol.*, **11**, 741.

— — (1966), 'The Early Development of the Eye in Staged Human Embryos', *Contrib. Embryol. Carnegie Instn*, **38**, 1.

PEARSON, A. A. (1980), 'The Development of the Eyelids', *J. Anat.*, **130**, 33.

— — JACOBSON, A. D., VAN CALCAR, R. J., and SAUTER, R. W. (1967), *The Development of the Ear*. Rochester, Minn.: American Academy of Ophthalmology and Otolaryngology.

PUJOL, R., and HILDING, D. (1973), 'Anatomy and Physiology of the Onset of Auditory Function', *Acta Otolaryngol.*, **76**, 1.

RUBEN, R. J., and RAPIN, I. (1980), 'Plasticity of the Developing Auditory System', *Ann. Otol. Rhinol. Laryngol.*, **89**, 303.

ZILLES, K. J. (1978), 'Ontogenesis of the Visual System', *Adv. Anat. Embryol. Cell. Biol.*, **54**, part 3.

185

CHAPTER 19

DEVELOPMENT OF THE DENTITION
(ODONTOGENESIS)

TEETH developed historically in primitive fishes from the adaptation of the ectodermal placoid scales overlying their jaws to form dermal denticles. This phylogenetic dermal origin of teeth is reflected in the embryonic development of human teeth, which although they develop submerged beneath the oral gingival epithelium, originate from ectodermal tissue. Teeth are derived from two of the primary germ layers, ectoderm and mesoderm, with a neural crest contribution. The enamel of teeth is derived from oral ectoderm and ectomesenchyme provides material for the dentine, pulp and cementum. The inner part of the periodontium is of neural crest origin, while the outer part is of mesodermal derivation.

Prior to any histological evidence of tooth development appearing, the alveolar nerves have grown into the jaws, and their branches form plexuses adjacent to sites of ectomesenchymal condensation, suggesting a possible neural inductive influence. Ectomesenchyme derived from the neural crest is the primary material of odontogenesis, since experimental ablation of neural crest tissue in amphibia has been shown to result in *anodontia* (absence of teeth).

Inductive interaction between neural crest tissue and pharyngeal endoderm, and subsequently with oral ectoderm is followed by a proliferation of the oral ectoderm which produces the first morphologically identifiable manifestation of tooth development, the *dental lamina*. The neural crest cells, in turn, are later induced to form the individual *dental papillae*, determining the future number of teeth (*Fig. 120*).

Potential odontogenic tissue can be identified as early as the 28th day of development (fertilization age) as areas of ectodermal epithelial thickening on the lateral margins of the stomodeum, at the same time that the oropharyngeal membrane disintegrates. The oral epithelium thickens on the inferolateral borders of the maxillary processes and on the superolateral borders of the mandibular arches where the two join to form the lateral margins of the stomodeum. Additional, and initially separate, odontogenic epithelium arises on the 35th day of development at the inferolateral borders of the frontonasal process, providing four separate sites of origin of odontogenic epithelium for the maxillary dentition. Accordingly, the anterior maxillary teeth would seem to be derived from the frontonasal process, and the posterior maxillary teeth from the

186

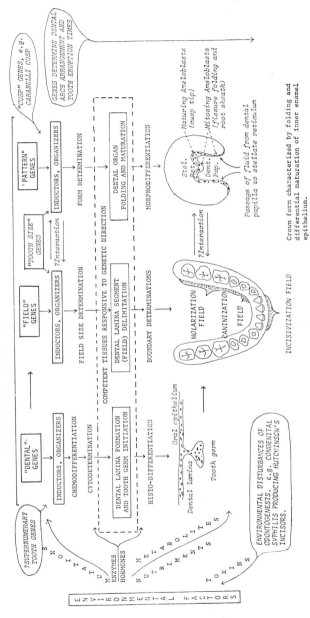

Fig. 120. Postulated mechanisms of odontogenesis. *(Copyright by Canadian Dental Association. Reprinted by permission.)*

187

maxillary processes. The mandibular dentition also develops four initial odontogenic sites in the mandibular arches, two on each side.

The four maxillary dental laminae coalesce on the 37th day, by which age the mandibular dental laminae have fused. The upper and lower dental laminae now form continuous horseshoe-shaped plates (*Fig. 121*). Local proliferations of the dental laminae are induced in a constant genetically determined sequence into the subjacent mesenchyme at locations corresponding to the dental papillae that are forming from neural crest cells. The positioning of teeth depends upon the discrete locations of competent mesenchyme responding to a continuous inductively active epithelium. The discontinuous distribution of nerve endings along the dental lamina and their possible influence on migrating neural crest cells accounts for ectomesenchymal localization beneath the oral epithelium with which interaction occurs. The ectodermal projections form the primordia of the *enamel organs*, and, together with the dental papillae, account for the subsequent submerged development of the teeth.

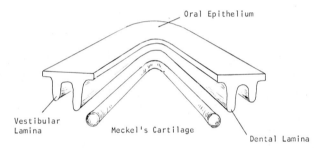

Fig. 121. Schematic representation of development of the mandibular vestibular and dental laminae.

Another, and later, subjacent proliferation of the oral epithelium occurs buccally and labially to the dental laminae and is known as the *vestibular lamina*. The vestibular laminae split the outer margins of the stomodeum into buccal segments that become the cheeks and lips and lingual segments in which the teeth and alveolar bone develop. Between the buccal and lingual segments there develops a sulcus, the *vestibule* of the mouth. Unsplit segments of the vestibular lamina remain as *frenula* (*sing. frenulum*).

Ten tooth germs, corresponding with the number of deciduous teeth, develop initially in each jaw. Each tooth germ consists of an enamel organ and a dental papilla surrounded by a *dental follicle* or *sac*. The dental papilla, of neural crest origin, and dental follicle of mesodermal origin, are the anlagen of the dental pulp and part of the periodontal apparatus respectively.

Each enamel organ during its growth and development alters its initially small *bud* shape by enlarging as a result of rapid rates of mitosis of the basal cells into a *cap* shape, and later cupping into a large *bell* shape, by which shapes three stages of enamel organ development are designated (*Fig. 122*). Concomitant with these morphological alterations, histodifferentiation is occurring within the enamel organ. Its external layer forms the *outer enamel epithelium*, a layer of cuboidal cells subjacent to the developing follicle.

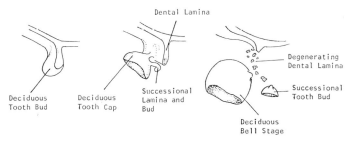

Fig. 122. The bud (*left*), cap (*middle*), and bell (*right*) stages of tooth development.

The *stellate reticulum*, composed of stellate cells set in a fluid matrix, constitutes the central bulk of the early enamel organ. The indented inner layer, lining the dental papilla, forms the *inner enamel epithelium*, part of which differentiates into the transient secretory columnar ameloblasts responsible for enamel formation. Lining a portion of the stellate reticular surface of the inner enamel epithelium is a squamous cellular condensation, the *stratum intermedium*, that probably assists enamel formation by the ameloblasts. The recurrent continuity of the inner and outer enamel epithelia at the *cervical loop* elongates into *Hertwig's epithelial root sheath*, that, by enclosing more and more of the dental papilla, outlines the root(s) of the tooth (*Fig. 123*). The number of roots of a tooth is determined by the subdivision, or lack thereof, of the root sheath into one, two, or three compartments.

The inner enamel epithelium interacts with the ectomesenchymal cells of the dental papilla whose peripheral cells differentiate into *odontoblasts*. The formation of dentine by the odontoblasts precedes, and is necessary for, the further induction of ameloblasts to produce enamel. The inner enamel epithelium of the root sheath induces odontoblast formation, but lacking a stratum intermedium, fails

189

to differentiate itself into enamel-forming ameloblasts, accounting for the absence of enamel from the roots. Where the outer enamel epithelium of the root sheath disintegrates cementum forms on the adjacent dentine. The fibres in the initial cementum are derived entirely from fibres of the pre-existing dental follicle that form the first principal fibres of the periodontal ligament.

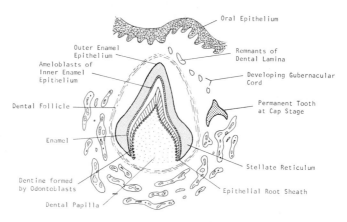

Fig. 123. Enamel organ of deciduous tooth in bony crypt.

The ameloblasts of the inner enamel epithelium lying adjacent to the odontoblasts together form a bilaminar amelodentinal membrane. The lengthening of this membrane by mitosis is under genetic control, and varies among the tooth germs in different areas. By the different foldings of the bilaminar membrane dictated by unknown factors residing in the underlying ectomesenchymal dental papilla the varying shapes of incisors, canines, premolars and molars are determined. The confined space of the dental follicle imposes foldings upon the lengthening amelodentinal membrane. These folds determine the form and sites of the cusps and grooves of the individual teeth. The folded amelodentinal membrane provides the template for the future shape of the crown of a tooth, which is elaborated upon by the subsequent deposition of enamel and dentine in opposite directions upon the bilaminar membrane. The ameloblasts secrete enamel rods or prisms as they retreat from the membrane, while the odontoblasts secrete the matrix of the pre-dentine, which later calcifies into dentine. Dentine deposition is a continuous process throughout life. The dental papilla converts into the dental pulp by histodifferentiation; the peripheral cells into odontoblasts, the remaining cells into fibroblasts. Enamel

190

formation is restricted to the pre-eruptive phase of odontogenesis and ends with the deposition of an organic layer, the *primary enamel cuticle*. The enamel organ flattens after deposition of the primary enamel cuticle. The inner and outer enamel epithelia together with the remains of the stratum intermedium form the *reduced enamel epithelium*. The reduced enamel epithelium later fuses with the overlying oral mucous membrane to initiate the pathway for eruption (*Fig. 124*).

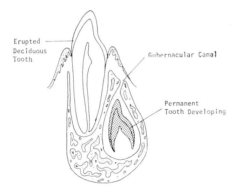

Erupted Deciduous Tooth

Gubernacular Canal

Permanent Tooth Developing

Fig. 124. Relationship of deciduous and permanent teeth in infancy.

Meanwhile, the mesenchyme surrounding the dental follicles becomes ossified, forming bony crypts in which the teeth develop, and from which they are later to erupt. An investing mesenchymal layer of the dental follicle adjacent to the cementum differentiates into the inner layer of the periodontal ligament by the development of collagen fibres. These fibres are already organized into inner, outer and intermediate layers between cementum and bone. The periodontal ligament is the medium through which orthodontic tooth movement is effected. The reorganization of the attachment apparatus, comprising cementum, periodontal fibres, and alveolar bone, following tooth movement, is a basic requisite to successful orthodontic treatment.

The anterior deciduous (incisor, canine, and first molar) tooth germs develop first, at the 6th week of life, while the second deciduous molar germs first appear at the 7th week. The anterior permanent (incisor, canine, and premolar) tooth germs bud from the lingual side of the corresponding deciduous enamel organs, while the second deciduous molar and permanent molar tooth germs develop directly from a backward extension of the dental lamina. The germs

191

of the first permanent molars initially develop at about the 16th week i.u., while those of the second and third permanent molars do not appear until after birth. Completion of permanent tooth formation does not take place until several years after birth, and in the case of the third molars, root formation is not completed until about the 21st year of age. In this respect, teeth have the most prolonged chronology of development of any set of organs in the body.

Tooth Eruption

The mechanisms by which teeth erupt have not been entirely elucidated, and a number of processes have been proposed to explain the movement of teeth from their crypts into the oral cavity. The elongation of the root of a tooth during its development, and the growth of the pulp within it while the apical foramen is wide open, are likely to be sources of at least part of the eruptive force. The deposition of cementum upon the surface of the root would provide some slight eruptive movement once root formation was completed. The path of eruption ahead of the crown of a tooth would be guided by the remnants of the attachments of the dental follicle to the oral epithelium from which it originated (gubernacular cords). Blood-pressure surrounding the root of a tooth and changes in the vascularity of the periodontal tissues have been implicated as eruptive forces.

A form of 'functional matrix' activity implicating an interplay between the periodontal ligament and the hard tissues has also been postulated in tooth eruption. The proliferating connective tissue of the periodontal ligament, or accumulation of periodontal tissue fluids resulting from increased vascular permeability would tend to separate tooth and bone, thereby providing an eruptive force. An inflamed, oedematous periodontal ligament pushes a tooth out of its socket, although this pathological phenomenon may not be strictly comparable to physiological eruption.

Another theory of tooth eruption suggests that contraction of the obliquely orientated collagen fibres of the periodontal ligament produces a 'pulling' force resulting in tooth eruption, in contrast to most of the 'pushing' forces indicated above (*Fig. 125*). The traction of the periodontal ligament has been attributed to contraction of fibroblasts. The presumed contraction of the fibroblasts of periodontal connective tissues has been likened to the contraction of scar tissue during wound healing. Contractile capabilities have been attributed to the fibroblasts of the periodontal and cicatricial connective tissues.

It is possible that tooth eruption is the result of the combination of a number of factors operating concomitantly or at different times during a tooth's period of eruption. The absence of any one of the erupting factors may be possibly compensated for by the activity of alternative factors. Tooth eruption appears to be an intermittent rather than a continuous process.* There are alternating stages of movement and equilibrium during eruption, concomitant with phases of general body growth spurts and quiescence. Individual post-eruptive tooth movement, producing migration and hyper-eruption, is subject to local factors of mastication or tooth disuse. The net eruptive force (eruption minus resistance) of a tooth is quite small, of the order of 5 grams of pressure.

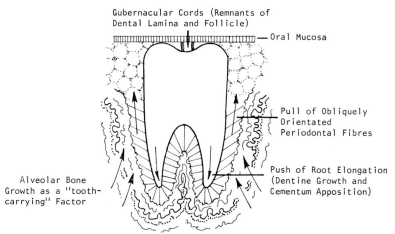

Fig. 125. Schematic synopsis of some various possible factors operating during tooth eruption.

The eruption of the molar teeth is combined with their mesial drift which ensures their contact with the anterior teeth, and their interproximal contact with one another when erupted. This tendency to mesial drift during eruption would account also for the frequently observed phenomenon of mesial impaction of unerupted teeth, in which the forward movement has occurred to a greater extent than the eruptive (upward or downward) movement. Protrusion of the anterior teeth may contribute to a dentally prognathic facial profile, while vertical tooth eruption compensates for loss of facial height resulting from attritional wear of the occlusal surfaces of teeth.

The regular sequence of eruption of teeth suggests that it is under

*Teeth that are continuously growing, e.g. the incisors of rodents, erupt continuously throughout life.

Table II.—CHRONOLOGY OF DEVELOPMENT AND ERUPTION OF TEETH

All dates postnatal, except where designated intrauterine (i.u.)

TOOTH	TOOTH GERM COMPLETED	CALCIFICATION COMMENCES	CROWN COMPLETED	ERUPTION IN MOUTH	ROOT COMPLETED
Deciduous					
Incisors		3–4 months i.u.	2–4 months	6–8 months	$1\frac{1}{2}$–2 years
Canines	12–16 weeks i.u.	5 months i.u.	9 months	16–20 months	$2\frac{1}{2}$–3 years
1st Molars		5 months i.u.	6 months	12–15 months	2–$2\frac{1}{2}$ years
2nd Molars		6–7 months i.u.	11–12 months	20–30 months	3 years
Permanent					
Central Incisors	30 weeks i.u.	3–4 months	4–5 years	Max.: 7–9 years Mand.: 6–8 years	9–10 years
Lateral Incisors	32 weeks i.u.	Max.: 10–12 months Mand.: 3–4 months	4–5 years	7–9 years	10–11 years
Canines	30 weeks i.u.	4–5 months	6–7 years	Max.: 11–12 years Mand.: 9–10 years	12–15 years
1st Premolars	30 weeks i.u.	$1\frac{1}{2}$–2 years	5–6 years	10–12 years	12–13 years
2nd Premolars	31 weeks i.u.	2–$2\frac{1}{2}$ years	6–7 years	10–12 years	12–14 years
1st Molars	24 weeks i.u.	Birth	$2\frac{1}{2}$–3 years	6–7 years	9–10 years
2nd Molars	6 months	$2\frac{1}{2}$–3 years	7–8 years	12–13 years	14–16 years
3rd Molars	6 years	7–10 years	12–16 years	17–21 years	18–25 years

194

genetic control. Considerable variation of the ages of tooth eruption does occur between individuals. Tooth eruption is highly subject to nutritional, hormonal, and disease conditions. Disturbances of the 'normal' sequence and ages of tooth eruption are contributory factors to the development of dental malocclusion, and consequently are of significance to orthodontists.

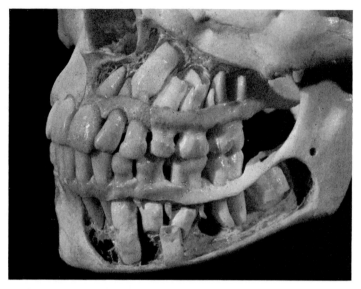

Fig. 126. The mixed deciduous and permanent dentition dissected in the skull of an 8-year-old child. Note the location of the unerupted permanent teeth in the bodies of the maxilla and mandible.

At birth, the jaws contain the partially calcified crowns of the 20 deciduous teeth, and the beginning of calcification of the first permanent molars (*Table II*). Eruption of the deciduous dentition, beginning on the average at $7\frac{1}{2}$ months of age, terminates on an average by 29 months of age. Dental eruption is then quiescent for nearly 4 years when, at the age of 6, the two jaws contain a greater number of teeth than at any other time. At this age, the jaws contain 48 teeth crammed between the orbits and nasal cavity and filling the body of the mandible (*Fig. 126*). Beginning at 6 years of age, all 8 deciduous incisors are lost and 12 permanent teeth erupt within a 2-year period. After this extreme activity, eruption is quiescent until $10\frac{1}{2}$ years of age, when the remaining 12 deciduous teeth are lost, and 16 permanent teeth all erupt within an 18-month period. The 6-year

195

period of the mixed dentition, ages 6 to 12 years, is the most complicated period of dental development and the one in which the development of malocclusion is most likely to occur. A long and variable
period (3–7 years) of quiescence follows before eruption of the 4
third molars completes the dentition. The third molars do not begin
calcifying until the 9th year of age, and their eruption from the 16th
year onwards heralds the completion of dentofacial growth and
development.

The permanent molars all originate from identical sites in each
quadrant of the jaw. The upper three molars originate from the
maxillary tuberosity of each side, while the lower three molars of
each side originate within the ascending ramus of the mandible.
The first and second molars migrate forward from their sites of
origin into the alveolar bone of the maxilla or mandible, from which
they erupt to meet their antagonists.

The vacating by the first permanent molars of their sites of origin
by 3 years of age allows space for the second molars to begin their
development in the same relative location. After the second molars
have migrated forwards by the 9th year of age, the vacated spaces
allow the third molars to begin their development. Failure of
adequate continued bone growth of the jaws during this period, for
either genetic or environmental reasons, precludes adequate space
for full eruption of all the permanent teeth, resulting in maleruption,
partially impacted eruption, or non-eruption of the last teeth to
occupy the space, viz., the third molars.

All the teeth in the jaws are carried downwards, forwards, and
laterally as the face expands, except for the central incisors, which
maintain their proximity to the median plane. The faster rate of
tooth eruption is superimposed upon this slower bone movement,
which combination of movements determines dental and gnatho-
skeletal growth patterns. The continual tendency of the teeth to
erupt and migrate means that this mechanism is constantly compensating for attritional wear of teeth to stabilize the vertical dimension
of the face. The maintenance of dental occlusion is a combination
of bone remodelling and tooth eruption that reflect the neuromuscular actions of the orofacial apparatus.

SELECTED BIBLIOGRAPHY

BARNETT, E. M., and MEHTA, J. D. (1970), 'Oral Growth Stages—The Keys
to Guiding Occlusal Development', J. Am. dent. Ass. 81, 1360.
BRADY, C. L., BROWNE, R. M., CALVERLEY, B. C., MARSLAND, E. A., and
WHITEHEAD, F. I. H. (1970), 'Symposium on Odontogenic Epithelium',
Br. J. oral Surg., 8, 1.

BURDI, A. R., GARN, S. M., and MILLER, R. L. (1970), 'Developmental Advancement of the Male Dentition in the First Trimester', *J. dent. Res.*, **49**, 889.

BUTLER, P. M., and JOYSEY, K. A. (Ed.) (1978), *Development, Function and Evolution of Teeth*, London: Academic Press.

CARLSEN, O. (1967), 'Odontogenetic Morphology', *Odont. Tidsk.*, **75**, 499.

CLINCH, L. (1966), 'Symposium on Aspects of the Dental Development of the Child (1) The Development of the Deciduous and Mixed Dentitions', *Dent. Practnr dent. Rec.*, **17**, 135.

DICKSON, G. C. (1970), 'The Natural History of Malocclusion', *Ibid.*, **20**, 216.

GARN, S. M., BURDI, A. R., MILLER, R. L., and NAGY, J. M. (1970), 'Prenatal Dental Development as a Reference Standard for Embryologic Status', *J. dent. Res.*, **49**, 894.

HAAVIKKO, K. (1970), 'The Formation and the Alveolar and Clinical Eruption of the Permanent Teeth', *Suom. HammaslääkSeur. Toim.*, **66**, 103.

HIXON, E. H., (1971), 'Growth of the Dentition and its Supporting Structure', *J. Am. dent. Ass.* **82**, 782.

INFANTE, P. F., and OWEN, G. M. (1973), 'Relation of Chronology of Deciduous Tooth Emergence to Height, Weight and Head Circumference in Children', *Archs oral Biol.*, **18**, 1411.

KOLLAR, E. J., and LUMSDEN, A. G. S. (1979), 'The Role of Innervation During Induction and Pattern Formation', *J. Biol. Bucc.*, **7**, 49.

KRAUS, B. S., and JORDAN, R. E. (1965), *The Human Dentition before Birth*. Philadelphia: Lea & Febiger.

LUNT, R. C., and LAW, D. B. (1974a), 'A Review of the Chronology of Calcification of Deciduous Teeth', *J. Am. dent. Ass.*, **89**, 599.

— — — — (1974b), 'A Review of the Chronology of Eruption of Deciduous Teeth', *Ibid.*, **89**, 872.

MCNAMARA, J. A. (Ed.) (1977), *The Biology of Occlusal Development*, Monograph 7, Craniofacial Growth Series. Center for Human Growth and Development. Ann Arbor: University of Michigan.

MATTHIESSEN, M. E., and RØMERT, P. (1980), 'Ultrastructure of the Human Enamel Organ', *Calc. Tiss. Res.*, **205**, 361.

MOORREES, C. F. A. (1959), *The Dentition of the Growing Child.* 1–245. Cambridge: Harvard Univ. Press.

MOYERS, R. E. (1973), *Handbook of Orthodontics*, 3rd ed. Chicago: Year Book Medical.

NERY, E. B., KRAUS, B. S., and CROUP, M. (1970), 'Timing and Topography of Early Human Tooth Development', *Archs oral Biol.*, **15**, 1315.

PEARSON, A. A. (1977), 'The Early Innervation of the Developing Deciduous Teeth', *J. Anat.*, **123**, 563.

POOLE, D. F. G., and STACK, M. V. (Ed.) (1976), *The Eruption and Occlusion of Teeth*. London: Butterworth.

SCOTT, J. H., and SYMONS, N. B. B. (1977), *Introduction to Dental Anatomy*, 8th ed. Edinburgh: Churchill Livingstone.

SLAVKIN, H. C. (1974), 'Embryonic Tooth Formation', *Oral Sciences Reviews*, No. 4. Copenhagen: Munksgaard.

SLAVKIN and BAVETTA, L. A. (1968), 'Odontogenic Epithelial-Mesenchymal Interactions in Vitro', *J. dent. Res.*, **47,** 779.

— — — — (1972), *Developmental Aspects of Oral Biology.* New York: Academic Press.

SPERBER, G. H. (1967), 'Genetic Mechanisms and Anomalies in Odontogenesis', *J. Can. dent. Ass.*, **33,** 433.

TEN CATE, A. R. (1980), *Oral Histology: Development, Structure and Function.* St. Louis: Mosby.

— — MILLS, C., and SOLOMON, G. (1971), 'The Development of the Periodontium. A Transplantation and Autoradiographic Study', *Anat. Rec.*, **170,** 365.

TONGE, C. H. (1969), 'The Time-structure Relationship of Tooth Development in Human Embryogenesis', *J. dent. Res.*, **48,** 745.

VAN DER LINDEN, F. P. G. M., and DUTERLOO, H. S. (1976), *Development of the Human Dentition.* Hagerstown, MD: Harper & Row.

INDEX

Page numbers appearing in **bold** type indicate major descriptions